Verbal Questioning Skills

For Kinesiologists

Jane Thurnell-Read

My thanks to John Payne for his support while this book was being written, for his attention to detail with proof reading, and for his questioning of my questioning.

ISBN: 978-0-9542439-1-3

Published by:

Life-Work Potential Limited
Sea View House
Long Rock
Penzance
Cornwall
TR20 8JF
England

Tel: 01736 719030
Fax: 01736 719040
www.lifeworkpotential.com

Other books by the author:

Energy Mismatch
ISBN: 978-0-9542439-3-7, Life-Work Potential, 2004

Allergy A To Z
ISBN: 978-0-9542439-2-0, Life-Work Potential, 2005

Geopathic Stress
ISBN: 978-0-9542439-4-4 Life-Work Potential, 2006

Health Kinesiology: The Muscle Testing System That Talks To The Body
ISBN 978-0-9542439-6-8, Life-Work Potential Limited, 2009

Nutritional Testing For Kinesiologists And Dowsers
ISBN: 978-0-9542439-5-1, Life-Work Potential Limited, 2009

CONTENTS

INTRODUCTION

Asking verbal questions is one of the most useful skills for a kinesiologist to acquire – unfortunately it is also one of the most difficult.

More and more kinesiologists are now using verbal questioning for all or part of their work. Many kinesiologists who rely extensively on finger modes eventually find they run out of finger modes and so resort to the occasional verbal question. Some of the antagonism against verbal questioning voiced by some of the kinesiology community is to my mind clearly attributable to the fact that they have not been taught to ask precise verbal questions, nor had much experience of those who have.

Inexpertly asked verbal questions do not further the cause of kinesiology nor of healing. Correctly formulated verbal questions enhance any kinesiology practice and the well-being of clients fortunate enough to be exposed to this rigorous discipline.

If you have reservations, I suggest you start by studying this book, and then use verbal questioning in situations where you have a clear opportunity to verify your answers by monitoring what happens to your clients.

I first started when I was introduced to it by Dr Jimmy Scott. Jimmy Scott developed health kinesiology in the 1980's and is a master of verbal questioning. His teaching and insight started me on the long road (not yet completed) of honing my skills as a verbal questioner. Along that road I have made some spectacular mistakes.

Some years ago, when my sons were small, I was visiting my parents for a few days. One of the boys was being very obnoxious and trying everyone's patience, so I decided to do some work on him. His energy system insisted that the work had to be spread over two days. At the end of the first session I asked: "When will I notice a difference from the work I have done – will it be today?"

The answer was 'yes'. Further questioning indicated that the difference would be noticeable within a couple of hours. I was much relieved by this, but after a while my son's behaviour got worse and worse, and I was mystified because I had tested that I would notice a difference within a couple of hours. Eventually the penny dropped: I had assumed that 'difference' meant 'improvement'. Of course, I should have asked something like: "When will I notice the benefit / positive difference of the work I have done?"

On another occasion a client told me that there were reputed to be gold sovereigns in her very old house, hidden there by a long dead sea captain. She asked if I could help her find them. I didn't know if I could do this, but was interested enough to have a try. Using muscle testing I asked: "Is there any hidden treasure in this house?" The response was positive, and so, amid great excitement, we tested to find the exact spot. Finally we came to the conclusion that the treasure was under a large chest freezer in the basement. When the chest freezer was removed, hidden treasure was indeed found: a one-pound coin that had obviously rolled under there at some point! She did dig down into the earthen floor but found nothing further. My question had been about hidden treasure not about gold sovereigns. A more precise question would have been: "Are there any gold sovereigns buried in this house?"

I hope that you will use this book to improve your verbal questioning skills and to fast-forward your learning process on the back of my mistakes and insights.

This is a book for kinesiologists. Unlike most kinesiology books it does not teach you new procedures, important as these are. It is designed to help you develop confidence in your own ability to ask rigorous verbal questions in a wide range of situations. Whatever kinesiology you practice or are learning this will enhance that practice immeasurably.

Jane Thurnell-Read

For many of the examples in this book I have used situations involving flower remedies, affirmations and nutrition. I have deliberately done this, because I want this book to appeal to a wide range of kinesiologists. The questioning skills taught in this book have much wider implications and applications for the way in which you practice. Please adapt this information to the particular type of kinesiology you use.

BASIC CONSIDERATIONS

Systematic Questioning Versus Intuition

One of the aims of this book is to help you to ask questions systematically. Many people rely predominantly or solely on intuition. But this does not always work. Sometimes your intuition is just not working very well; this particularly tends to happen if you are tired or disturbed in your own life. It may also apply when you are working on emotional problems for a client that are similar to your own emotional issues.

The Importance Of Intention

Many kinesiologists seem to feel that they do not need to be rigorous in their work, because their good intention will carry them through. Undoubtedly many times you will get excellent results even when your questions are badly formed, but some energy systems will respond very precisely to the question as it is asked. Also, if your intention is to do sloppy work, (and this is your intention if you are not prepared to exercise the necessary self-discipline to learn how to ask rigorous questions), you will get sloppy, unsatisfactory results.

Tuning Into Universal Knowledge

Some practitioners and students do not feel they need to put a lot of effort into understanding scientific knowledge, because they believe they can tune into 'universal knowledge' for anything they do not know. I accept that some people can do this at least some of the time, but many students and practitioners get very poor results relying on this external source. Monitor the results of this type of work particularly carefully. After all, if it were that easy and reliable to tune into universal knowledge, we could all be brain surgeons as well as kinesiologists.

Pedantic Bodies

Some bodies are very literal in their interpretation of what you are saying. For example, look at this question:

- Do you need to take a flower remedy every day?

The muscle response from most people would be 'yes' if the person needed to take one or more flower remedies a day, but pedantic bodies may give the answer 'no' to this question if more than one flower remedy is required. Pedantic bodies often seem to be owned by pedantic personalities, so be on the look out for this. These clients really give us a chance to perfect our verbal questioning skills!

Silent Questioning

Silent questioning has several advantages:

- Clients cannot seek to influence the test results, as they do not know what questions are being asked.
- Asking silent questions is usually quicker than asking questions out loud.

The main disadvantage of it is that it allows sloppy questioning – when questions are not formulated out loud, some precision is lost.

Silent questioning also raises ethical questions about what questions should be asked. My own rule of thumb is that I will only ask questions silently that I would be prepared to tell the client immediately if they asked me what the question was that I had just asked.

Which Muscles To Use

You can use any muscle for verbal testing. I usually use the brachioradialis (in the forearm). Clients in general find this a very comfortable muscle to use, because when the client is lying down the upper arm is resting on the couch. It is also very easy to explain to the client how they need to position the arm for the test. Whichever muscle you choose use your normal techniques or checks to ensure that the muscle is responding predictably.

At times you will be doing an extensive amount of verbal questioning so it is important to use as light a touch as possible, and to change muscles if the client experiences fatigue.

Which Muscle Response Means 'Yes' And Which Means 'No'?

In general a strong or locked muscle response indicates 'yes', and a spongy, weak or unlocked muscle response means 'no'.

Using Statements Rather Than Questions

Some kinesiologists prefer to use statements rather than verbal questions. As I am a health kinesiologist, I am used to using verbal questions, but the explanations in this book can be adapted if you prefer to use statements. You will probably notice in some of the examples that I phrase the question by making a statement and then adding 'Is this correct?' on the end.

Initial Balance

Many practitioners work without checking that the energy system is balanced. This clearly works: clients do get better. Most of these practitioners are using finger modes, reflex points and challenging to establish what is needed. My experience suggests that having the energy system balanced is more critical when using verbal questioning. Many kinesiologies have pre-checks, and health kinesiology offers a series of checks for different aspects of balance as a preliminary to undertaking any work.

Protective Devices

Sometimes clients will come in wearing a protective device, such as a programmed crystal or something to protect against electro-magnetic pollution. It is possible that such a device will interfere with the testing by masking some stressor(s). If this were the case, you would get a false picture from your testing. There are two possibilities; you can:

-   Ask the client to remove the device.
-   Check whether or not the device will interfere with the testing.

The first option is straightforward. In order to test for the second option, you have to take the device off, because if it were a problem it might interfere with the answer to the question asking if it is a problem! In general, as the client is going to have to remove it to test whether it needs removing, it is easier just to ask them to remove it for the session anyway. However, if you did want to check, you would get them to remove the item and then ask:

-   Is there any reason why you should not wear the crystal during the session?

You might also want to test if the device is beneficial for the client. You can do that by employing similar questions to the ones discussed in the section on questioning procedures where clients are already taking supplements.

When Clients Are Pregnant, Extremely Ill Or On Powerful Medication

Many practitioners are nervous about working on people like this, because they are concerned about doing more harm than good, even though they know that muscle testing should take care of this. I tend to preface questions with the phrase 'bearing in mind', when I am working in a situation of this sort, e.g.

- Bearing in mind that you are six months pregnant, would it be appropriate for us to work together?
- Bearing in mind that you are on tablets for your high blood pressure, would it be appropriate to carry out technique X?
- Bearing in mind that you are seriously ill with colon cancer, would it be appropriate for you to take this supplement?

Although this is unnecessary, it does give the client (and me!) an extra layer of confidence.

Enlisting The Client's Help

Sometimes it speeds things up if you ask the client for suggestions, but sometimes their suggestions are misleading, or they forget about something important.

In one session I was trying to locate a scar. I asked the client where she had scars on her body, but none of these tested as being the scar that needed work at that moment. So I asked her what other scars she had. She was adamant that she did not have any more scars. I persisted, but she was still insistent too. Eventually I scanned her body to find the illusive scar. Testing said it was on her left lower arm and sure enough I found a two-inch scar there. Even when I pointed it out to her she told me she had no knowledge of it.

With another client I established that I needed a list of five ex-girlfriends. I asked him for the names of all his ex-girlfriends and tested each in turn, and we found four of them this way. He told me that he had not had any other girlfriends, so I checked again that I needed a fifth name. Then I had to wait while he thought about his past. Suddenly he said: "Of course, I've left out my first ever girlfriend." Testing confirmed this was the missing woman.

Appropriate Is An Appropriate Word To Use!

I use 'appropriate' a lot when asking verbal questions. It is easy to become slipshod and ask questions using 'can' instead, e.g.

- Can you eat wheat?

This means: Are you able to eat wheat? and can lead to a misleading answer if the body says 'yes', (because you are able to eat wheat as you have teeth, know how to eat, etc.) A better question is:

- Is it appropriate for you to eat wheat?

The word 'beneficial' is also useful, e.g.

- Would it be beneficial for you to eat wheat?

Is this OK?

Using OK in verbal questioning is rarely OK! For example, what does it mean to ask:

- Is it OK for you to eat potatoes?

Surely we are not interested in what is OK, but in what is best or optimal for the client.

Instead we might want to ask one of these questions:

- Is it appropriate for you to eat potatoes?
- Would you significantly benefit in health terms from eating potatoes?

What is 'It'?

Whenever I use the word 'it' in a verbal question I always double-check the question, because 'it' implies a singular amount, but you may not have established that it is just one. For example:

- Would it be appropriate for you to take Bach Flower Remedies? Yes
- Is it Rock Rose?

In these two questions you have moved from the plural to the singular without establishing that this is correct. Written down like this, it looks improbable that you would make such a mistake, but I have seen it happen repeatedly when students are learning verbal questioning skills.

Is There An Easier / Cheaper / Quicker Way To Do This?

Sometimes new students and practitioners want to ask this question if they come up with something that is a problem in some way for the client, but this is really a superfluous question – if there were an easier / cheaper / quicker way to achieve the same result the energy system would have come up with that initially. It may be possible to offer *less effective* alternatives. A good way to evaluate these is by using indexes (see later).

Is This Precise Enough?

Sometimes the energy system wants absolute precision, and sometimes it wants a range to be given. For example, if you are working out the time in the day at which a client should perform a visualisation, it might be vitally important for some energetic reason that it starts at exactly 8.00 p.m. every night. On the other hand it might not matter that much, as long as it is started between 7.45 p.m. and 8.15 p.m., or the energy system may not want the instructions to be too precise, because this will set up unnecessary stress on the person. Do not guess or make an assumption as to which is correct, test:

- So you need to start your visualisation between 7.45 p.m. and 8. 15 p.m.? Yes
- Is that precise enough? Yes

Another situation in which this may occur is when you are checking quantities of food, so the energy system may be quite happy with the instruction 'eat 15-20 almonds a day' or it may want it to be 'eat 17 almonds a day'. Once again you need to test for how precise you need to be.

Asking Check Questions

It is important to build checks into your questioning. Confirmatory questions are extremely important. There are many times when you may believe you have looked at all the options and covered all the possibilities, but you have not done so. Even when you are very experienced at asking verbal questions, this will still happen. There are three main ways of doing this:

- Asking a general check question.
- Asking a summarising question.
- Asking an opposing question.

There are many different ways you can phrase general check questions, but I usually use:

- Is everything correct so far?

It is very important when you ask this question to test carefully, and not just assume that the reply will be 'yes'. Be a little humble and be prepared to have got something wrong.

Asking a summarising question is particularly useful when you are coming up with something very complicated:

- So, you need to touch the tip of your nose with the thumb of your left hand while you think the words 'I am strong', and at the same time you must look at the blue shirt you're wearing. Is that completely correct?

The third way of asking check questions is to ask opposing questions, where you expect the answer 'yes' to one and 'no' to the other:

- Is everything correct so far?
- Do I need to change anything?

or

- For optimum health do you need to avoid all wheat?
- It is appropriate for you to eat some wheat?

Asking opposing questions can also be helpful in stopping you making an assumption. Look at this question:

- Do the carrots need to be eaten raw? No

If you are not careful, you could assume from this that the carrots must be eaten cooked, but let's ask the opposing question:

- Do the carrots need to be eaten cooked?

If you get 'yes' to this, then you know that the carrots should not be eaten raw. However, if you get the answer 'no' to this, you know that it is not important whether the carrots are eaten raw or cooked.

Is There Anything Else We Need To Know About This?

This is an extremely important question that you will use, for example, when working out homework for the client. If you do not use this question, you can go on asking a lot of other questions, all of which have a negative answer. Let me give you an example of this. You have worked out that the client needs to say an affirmation 'I am happy and well', three times a day for the next six weeks. Then, rather than asking 'Is there anything else we need to know about this', you ask a whole additional series of questions:

- Does this need to be out loud? No
- So, this needs to be silent? No
- Oh, so it's not important whether it's said out loud or silently. Is that correct? Yes
- Does it matter where you are when you say the affirmation? No
- Is the exact time of day the affirmations are said important? No
- Is it important that you're on your own? No
- Is it important that other people are there? No
- So it doesn't matter whether you're on your own or with other people – is that correct? Yes

You can see how you can spend a lot of time asking questions that are not relevant. Asking the question 'Is there anything else we need to know about this?' can stop this process in its tracks. Obviously sometimes when you ask this question, you will get the answer 'yes'. In those cases you carry on and find another factor / component, and then once again ask if there is anything else you need to know. You keep doing this until you get the answer 'no' to the question asking if there is anything else.

Is It Important?

Sometimes, when you have already found some information for the
client, they will query some aspect of it. For example, you have
found that the client needs to drink eight glasses of water a day, and
the client might ask: "Should I drink that with meals?" You should
have concluded your previous questioning by asking if there is
anything else that you need to know, so you know that it does not
matter when the client drinks the water. Clients are not always
reassured by this explanation, so in these circumstances I often ask
a question such as:

- Is it important whether this water is drunk with or away
  from meals?

You will get the answer 'no' to this, but it seems to reassure clients
much more than the explanation does.

Conflicting Answers

Sometimes you will get apparently conflicting answers. There are
two reasons for this:

- Either you or the client is out of balance and so giving
  incorrect answers; it isalso possible that both of you are
  out of balance.
- You are making some assumption about the information
  that you have been given that is incorrect.

If I get conflicting answers, I usually try first to see if I am making
some wrong assumption. If I cannot find any, I run the normal pre-
checks I use to see if the client and I are balanced. If one of us is
out of balance, I correct this, and then establish how much of what I
have already found is correct. I usually ask about each component
of what I have found individually:

- Is it correct that you take vitamin C? Yes

- Is it correct that you take this once a day in the morning? Yes
- Etc.

If both you and the client are balanced, it is likely that you are making some assumptions about the information you have gained from the muscle testing. You need to think slowly and carefully about what *precise* questions you asked, and what the answers really meant.

Would This Be A Good Starting Point?

Sometimes, particularly when trying to find something complex, it is good to get a clue to point you in the right direction. Questions that might be appropriate, depending on the circumstances, include:

- Would the blood type diet be a good starting point?
- Would the discussion we had before we started this session be a good starting point?
- Would the Behavioural Barometer be a good starting point?
- Would my Louise Hay book give us a clue to the affirmation we are looking for?

Remember you are asking for a pointer to get you into the right direction to help you on your way. If you get 'yes' to the question about the blood type diet, for example, it does not mean that the client should follow the diet for their blood type in its entirety. You need to ask further questions to establish if this is the case, e.g.

- Do you follow it exactly?

If you got no to this, you need to find which aspects need to be changed.

Narrowing Items Down On A List

You may want to use a list for various reasons, e.g. to find a particular word, or type of procedure (also see What Do I do First? under Managing The Session). You could ask randomly till you hit on the correct one, or you could ask about each individually in turn starting at the top. Both of these methods would result in you eventually finding the correct item, but it could take a long time, so it is better to be systematic. One of the best ways to do this is to divide the page up, so you ask first about the top half of the list. If you get 'yes' to this you would divide that top half in half and ask about each of these sections. So, an example finding a word on a list might look like this:

- Is the exact word we are looking for on this list? Yes
- Is it one of these? (pointing to the top half of the list) No
- Is it one of these? (pointing to the bottom half of the list) Yes
- Is it between here and here? (pointing to the top half of the bottom half of the list) No
- Is it between here and here? (pointing to the bottom half of the bottom half of the list) Yes
- Is it one of these? (pointing to a few items) Yes
- Etc

One way of simplifying this further is to divide your list up into sections and name the sections. This is particularly appropriate for lists you use frequently. Then the session would look something like this:

- Is the one we are looking for in sections A to D? No
- In sections E to H? Yes
- In section E or F? No
- In section G or H? Yes
- Section G? Yes

If you have several pages rather than a single page, you would follow the same procedure, asking first about the first half and then about the second half. For example, if you had a list covering five pages, the beginning of the questioning might look like this:

- Is the item I am looking for on pages one to three? No
- Is the item on page four or five? Yes

Inadvertently Excluding The Mid Point

You must be careful in your questioning not to omit inadvertently the middle point. For example, look at these two questions:

- Is it before July? No
- Is it after July? No

You would get this if it were <u>in</u> July.

In the following example, you would need to move your finger slightly so that the middle word is included in either the 'above' or 'below' question, otherwise you will be excluding the middle word:

- Is it above this word on the list?
- Is it below this word on the list?

Alternatively, you could phrase these questions as:

- Is it this word or above on this list?
- Is it below this word on the list?

Testing For Something, But The Client Already Doing It

Sometimes something comes up in testing that the client is already doing. For example, in nutritional testing you could get that the person should avoid all dairy products or take a particular supplement, and they tell you that they are already doing this. You may think you have made a mistake, but often, when you question the client more closely, they will say that they have had doubts that it is the right thing to do, or that they have not been as strict as they should be about it lately, or that family members or friends have been criticising or mocking them for what they have been doing. The client's energy system is taking the opportunity of the questioning to reinforce the existing practice to ensure that the practice continues.

Activities

Sometimes you need to find an activity. It may be something the client needs to do during the session, or something they do afterwards.

Sometimes you have a good idea (based on intuition or on what has gone before) about the nature of the task. In this case, name the task and then ask:

- Would it be appropriate to use this task?

If you get 'yes', do not forget to ask the check question:

- Do we need to know anything more about this task?

If you have got everything exactly right, you will get 'yes' to the first question and 'no' to the second question. If you get 'yes' to both questions, this means that you have the correct basic task, but that you need to make some alterations to the way it is done. In this case the following general questions are appropriate to get you focussed in the right direction:

- Do we need to know something more about **how** this task is done?
- Do we need to know something more about **when** this task is done?
- Do we need to know something more about **where** this task is done?

If you get 'yes' to the first question, stop and establish exactly what the change is. Then ask:

- Do we need to know anything more about this task?

If you get 'no', ask the check question:

- Do we now have everything correct about this task?

You should get the answer 'yes' if you have got all the information you need. If you get 'no' you would then go on and ask the next question:

- Do we need to know something more about when this task is done?

This is getting complicated, so let me put this in a table for you:

	Question	*Answer*	*Action*
Question 1	Do we need to know something more about **how** this task is done?	yes	find out what it is, then go to Question 4
Question 1	Do we need to know something more about **how** this task is done?	no	go to Question 2

	Question	*Answer*	*Action*
Question 2	Do we need to know something more about **when** this task is done?	yes	find out what it is, then go to Question 4
Question 2	Do we need to know something more about **when** this task is done?	no	go to Question 3
Question 3	Do we need to know something more about **where** this task is done?	yes	find out what it is, then go to Question 4
Question 3	Do we need to know something more about **where** this task is done?	no	go to Question 4
Question 4	Do we have everything we need to know for this task?	yes	go to Question 5
Question 4	Do we have everything we need to know for this task?	no	recheck questions 1-3
Question 5	Is there anything else we need to know for this task?	yes	recheck
Question 5	Is there anything else we need to know for this task?	no	give the client the instruction

If it is not obvious what the activity is, you need to do some systematic questioning to narrow down the options. The main possibilities for the client are:

- Changing something about an existing activity (e.g. increasing the number of gym visits, changing the time that supplements are taken, etc.)
- Taking something (e.g. supplement, flower remedy, herbs, etc.)
- Doing something (e.g. exercise, sport, breathing exercise, affirmation, visualisation, etc.)
- Wearing something (e.g. a crystal, an energy device, a colour, etc.)
- Stopping some activity.

I include stopping some activity here otherwise it can tend to be overlooked.

Replacements

Quite often you will test for a reduction or cessation in some activity, e.g. eating a particular food, doing a particular activity, cooking with a particular type of utensil. One of the dangers of this is that the client might replace the activity with another activity that is equally bad or even more harmful, so it is important to address this in the questioning. For example, if you test that a client needs to reduce their intake of coffee to a maximum of two cups a day, it probably would not be a good thing for them to replace the missing cups with tea or alcohol. In these circumstances I usually ask the client what they would like to use as a replacement and test this. If this does not test as being suitable, I ask for another choice and keep on testing till I get a suitable substitute or better still a range of substitutes.

For example, testing has shown that a client must reduce their normal ten cups of coffee a day to a maximum of two a day. I then ask what they would like to replace it with, and they suggest tea:

- Would it be appropriate to replace some or all of the coffee with tea? Yes

- All of it? No
- More than one cup? No
- So, one cup of tea in addition to the two cups of coffee?
  Yes
  (I ask the client for other substitutes, and they suggest
  chamomile tea. I decide to ask a more general question
  first.)
- Would herb teas be a suitable replacement for some or all
  of the coffee? Yes
- Chamomile tea? Yes
- Would it be appropriate for all of it to be chamomile tea?
  No
- More than four cups? No
- Less than three cups? No
- Three cups? Yes
- Would it be appropriate to have other herbal teas? Yes

I would carry on the questioning until I establish all the
replacements that would be suitable. Where possible always give
the client several different options for the replacement.

Making Decisions Using Muscle Testing

Some kinesiologists use muscle testing to determine their choices
and actions in every day life. Before going on a train journey they
will test which train to take. They will test which clothes to buy,
which books to read, and so on. I feel this is an inappropriate use of
this wonderful skill. Part of life is taking responsibility for our
actions and making mistakes. Sometimes muscle testing can be
useful in helping you make choices. For example, if you suffer
from allergy problems you might want to use muscle testing to
establish what to eat before choosing a meal in a restaurant. But
allowing your whole life to be dictated by muscle testing removes
the growth potential of making decisions in the normal way.

FINDING THOUGHTS, WORDS & PHRASES

There are various reasons you may need to find a series of words or a topic, e.g. to establish the topic for ESR or to work out an affirmation or to give the client a specific phrase to think as part of a procedure.

Thinking Something/Thinking About Something

If thinking is involved in any procedure, it is important to be clear from the beginning if the client is thinking about something or thinking a specific word, phrase or sentence. If they are thinking about something, you need to find the general topic, and then the client thinks about different aspects of it as they see fit. If the client needs to think something, you need to find the specific word or words that they will think over and over again.

Whatever the client has to think it is important that the client is left to think without you explaining why you think it is significant. The client's energy system has chosen those particular words or this topic because they will trigger the right emotional and energetic response. If you explain what these mean to the client, you will be putting your interpretation on them, and this could trigger a whole series of emotions and feelings which are not correct for the client at that time.

How To Proceed

There are several different ways of finding thoughts, words and phrases:

- Intuition.
- Logical, working on what you know about the client.
- Using lists (discussed earlier).
- Starting from scratch and working systematically.

You will probably use all of these methods at different times depending on the circumstances.

How Many Words?

If the person has to think something specific, it is often useful to find out how many words are involved. When you ask this at the beginning, the question is simple, e.g.

- How many words are we looking for – at least two?

If you have already found some of the words, your question needs to be clear, as there are two different ways of finding the additional words. You can ask, for example:

- How many additional words are we looking for – at least four?

Or

- How many words do we have for this item in total – at least four?

Usually it is clearer to ask for additional words.

Which Word To Find First?

Having found the number of words involved it seems natural to start by finding the first word, but this is not always the fastest and easiest way to find all the words. For example, if you were working with a fellow kinesiologist and were looking for four words, and the answer was 'being a competent kinesiologist', finding the fourth word first would probably speed up the process. So you can ask some questions to establish which is the best word to find first, e.g.

- Is it best to find the first word first?

Is It To Do With X?

This question can be very useful, but I usually make it clearer by adding in the word 'obviously', e.g.

- Is this obviously to do with work?

So, for example, if the word you are looking for is 'mother', you would get 'no' as an answer to this question, even though ones relationship with ones mother can have an effect on work relationships. However, if the word you were trying to find was 'boss' or 'office' or 'promotion' or 'working', you would get the answer 'yes' to the question.

Using the word 'obviously' helps to keep the questioning focussed.

General Areas

When looking for words some general categories come up frequently so it is good to ask about these early on if it is appropriate. Common areas are:

- Emotions (e.g. fear, anger, love, happiness, misery, etc.)
- Feelings (e.g. hot, cold, shaky, in pain, etc.)
- Virtues and vices (e.g. honesty, integrity, truth, meanness, greed, adultery, etc.)
- Intellectual concepts (e.g. success, freedom, independence, etc.)
- Physical body (e.g. fat, thin, beautiful, sexy, stiff, in pain, ageing, etc.)

- Health / Ill health (e.g. healthy, fit, energetic, lively, vibrant, ill, unhealthy, dying, decrepit, etc.)
- Relationships (love, intimacy, tenderness, mother, relative, lover, etc.)
- Goals (e.g. future, purpose, intention, dreams, ideals, vision, objective, ambition, or a named goal of the client, etc.)
- Spirituality (e.g. God, spirit, enlightenment, religion, sin, etc.)

Do notice that these general categories are not mutually exclusive. For example, you could find the word 'love' through the emotions category and through the relationships category.

Using Grammar

If you learnt grammar at school, consider yourself lucky. If you did not (or you need a refresher course), look at appendix 2. Finding the grammatical structure of what the person thinks can help you quickly home in on suitable words or phrases. In fact some of health kinesiology's psychological techniques are categorised according to grammatical structures. This is not just for convenience, but because we believe that different grammatical structures have different energetic qualities.

It is easiest to show you the importance of grammar by giving some examples. Consider what the possibility could be if you wanted to find three words that the person needs to think. Here are some possibilities:

Using a conjunction such as 'and' or 'or', e.g.

- Happiness and success.
- Popular or respected.

Using a gerund, an adverb and an adjective, e.g.

- Being totally happy.
- Feeling happy now.

Using a prepositional phrase, e.g.

- In the middle.
- On the top.
- Without a clue.

Using a determiner and an adjective and a noun, e.g.

- A successful woman.
- A happy man.
- A competent kinesiologist.

There are these and other possibilities when you are looking for three words for the person to think, so it's good to start by asking what type of structure the words follow.

When you first start to ask questions in this way, you may find it cumbersome and slow, but gradually your skill will improve, and you will find this a quick way to get you started on finding the words you need.

If your grammar knowledge is not up to categorising words like this, spend some time studying appendix 2. You can also ask by giving examples, e.g.

- Is the structure similar to *a successful woman* / *a happy employee* / *a knowledgeable person?*

When asking this question, you are not asking if one of these phrases is correct, but simply if the correct words follow the same form. For example, you would get 'yes' if the phrase you were looking for were 'a lonely wife'.

You may see the point of asking questions about the grammatical structure of the thought, when you have several words to find, but it can also be useful when you have a single word to find. I have had several clients who have had to think words such as 'I' or 'myself' or 'them' or 'if' or 'when'. These sorts of items can be very difficult to find unless you ask questions such as:

- Is the word I'm looking for a pronoun? (e.g. me, them, us, why, when, etc.)
- Is the word I'm looking for a conjunction? (e.g. if, as, because, etc.)

The Most Appropriate Way To Find Something

Interestingly the easiest way to find something is sometimes not the most appropriate. This seems to occur particularly when you are trying to find psychological items. The item may well be on a list that you use frequently, but the energy system may gain something from a search that does not involve a list. So, for example, finding the word 'rage' on a list may be very different energetically from finding 'rage' via the following questions:

- Is the word we are looking for an emotion? Yes
- Is it a negative emotion? Yes
- Is it 'fear' or a word like that? No
- Is it 'anger' or a word like that? Yes
- Is it anger? No
- Is it less intense than anger? No
- Is it more intense than anger? Yes
- Is it fury? No
- Is it rage? Yes

Doing it this way, particularly out loud, seems to give a whole hinterland of associations, and so can make the procedure much deeper, richer and more significant for the client.

Synonyms/Clues

A synonym is a word that means the same as another word, so, for example, ill and unhealthy are classified as synonyms. Clues are not synonyms, but may be words that mean the opposite, or associated words. Here is an example:

- Is 'fat' a clue to the word we are looking for? Yes

The possibilities here are now numerous:

- The word could be 'fat' itself.
- The word could be a synonym for fat, e.g. obese, large, overweight, etc.
- The word could be an opposite of fat, e.g. thin, slim, slender, etc.
- The word could be associated with the word fat, e.g. diet / dieting, indulgence, abstinence, etc.

So questioning might look like this:

- Is the word actually 'fat'? No
- Is it a synonym of fat? No
- Is it an opposite of fat? Yes
- Is it slim? No
- Is it thin? Yes

Sometimes You Already have The Word You Are Looking For

Sometimes I have had egg on my face from missing the obvious, e.g.

- Is this a positive word? Yes

Once I spent a long time looking for this one before I found that the word was 'positive'.

On another occasion I was looking for a phrase and I had got as far as finding that it was 'fear of ....' Questioning had established that I was looking for one more word. Much to my embarrassment it took me a long time to establish that the word I was looking for was 'fear' – the phrase was 'fear of fear'. Since then I have had phrases like 'knowing knowledge', 'accepting acceptance', living life' and 'suffering suffering' come up for clients. Once you are aware of these types of possibilities such items are not that difficult to find.

Finding A Category Of People

Sometimes you need to find a category of people because, for example, the client needs to think about that during a kinesiology procedure, or as part of an affirmation, e.g. my work colleagues, people who are older than me, men, etc. Having established that you are looking for a category of people, you can next ask about what type of category in order to narrow down the options, e.g.

- Is this a gender category? (e.g. men, women, beautiful women, men who are cleverer than I am, etc.)
- Is this a relationship category? (e.g. sisters, siblings, my older cousins, parents, boyfriends, women I fancy, etc.)
- Is this a work category? (e.g. colleagues, customers, superiors)
- Is this an authority category? (e.g. police, bank managers, bosses, officials, etc.)

Once you have the category type you can usually find the words more easily.

Finding A Named Person

Sometimes rather than a category of people, you are looking for a named person, e.g. my mother, Anna, Susan and Peter, Uncle David, etc. Because these are often relatives, the first question you might want to ask is:

- Is this a relative?

In asking this question you are asking about both blood relatives and relatives by adoption or marriage. If you get 'yes' to this question, the next question would be:

- Is this a blood relative?

But this may be a can of worms, as the client may consider someone a blood relative who is not (because of adultery or adoption). So, I usually ask the question more bluntly:

- Are we looking for a blood relative, as that term is understood?

Sometimes it would not be appropriate to say this. In these situations I ask the simple question but have it clearly in mind that I am implying the more exact question.

If it is not a relative try these:

- Current or previous boyfriends/girl friends.
- Friends.
- Client's 'heroes', e.g. a sporting hero or a celebrity.
- Work colleagues / bosses

The client may have to think about someone for a variety of reasons. For example the client may have a difficult relationship with the named person, but it could equally be that the client admires some quality of the named person, or that they are symbolic in some other way. As a child my mother used to say to me: "Why can't you be like Margot?" – a neighbour's daughter who was always neat, tidy and obedient. When I think about Margot, I think about how in some ways I do not meet my mother's expectations of what she wanted her daughter to be.

Using Swear Words, Childish Words, Personal Words Or Specialist Terminology

Sometimes a word is difficult to find because it is a swear word, and such words often seem inappropriate in your communication with a client. On testing, one client had to think a specific swear word. I was very surprised because she seemed such a proper lady. When I explained this to her, she went bright red and told me that it was a word she used when she was on her own and was irritated with people.

Once I had to think a phrase for a correction on myself. Testing eventually produced 'doing 'ard things'. My energy system was very insistent; I must think the word 'ard not the word hard. Thinking it like this took me back to being a very small child, who sometimes found the world overwhelming. This produced a very different energy experience from thinking 'doing hard things', which would lead me to a much more adult experience.

Clients may also need words to do with their particular religious beliefs, their technical expertise, terms of endearment they use for those they love, or childhood names for body parts, etc. In these cases you will need to seek some active help from the client to establish the item.

Sometimes it is obvious that you are looking for a word to do with the person's religious beliefs or with their work, but not always. If I start to have difficulty find a word, I might ask the question:

- Is this a word that I am familiar with?

If I get the answer 'no', I have to enlist the client's help to track down the word.

Positive / Negative / Neutral

Some words are clearly positive or negative, e.g. hatred or selfishness, but others are more difficult to categorise. I categorise 'anger' as negative, because in general it is recognised as a negative word. What about words like 'me', 'myself' and 'them'? I categorise these as 'neutral'. Some words are even more problematic. Is 'soft' a negative or positive word? You might say it depends on the context, and you would be right, but for the purpose of verbal questioning you need to categorise it somehow.

In the final analysis it does not matter how you categorise words, as long as you do it consistently, so that if you get a 'yes' to *Is this a positive word?* you know whether 'soft', 'myself' etc. are now possibilities or have been excluded.

Basic Emotions And Their Spectrum

It is often said that the four basic human emotions are fear, sadness, happiness and anger, but some anthropological research has suggested that there are two additional emotions, making six in all:

- Fear
- Sadness
- Happiness
- Anger
- Sympathy
- Disgust

Lester Levenson uses the following categories of emotions in his work:

- Apathy
- Grief
- Fear
- Lust
- Anger
- Pride

- Courageousness
- Acceptance
- Peace

Another categorisation from Silvan S Tomkins is:

- Anger
- Interest
- Contempt
- Disgust
- Distress
- Fear
- Joy
- Shame
- Surprise

W Parrott defines six primary emotions:

- Love
- Joy
- Surprise
- Anger
- Sadness
- Fear

and then has secondary emotions linked to each of these categories, and then tertiary emotions linked to each of the secondary categories.

Whichever categorisation you use, these 'basic' emotions give you a starting point to finding the actual emotion involved, but don't forget the emotion you are looking for could be the basic one you have already identified. If it is not the basic emotion, you need to find an emotion that falls into that 'family'. So, for example fear words include anxiety, terror, shyness, panic, distress, etc. Looking at these words you can see that some are more intense than others, e.g. terror is stronger than fear, whereas anxiety is less intense than fear. This concept can aid you in finding the actual word you are looking for. The questioning might look like this:

- Are we looking for one of the anger emotions? Yes
- Is it anger? No
- Is it stronger than anger? No
- Is it weaker than anger? Yes
- Is it impatience? No
- Is it irritation? Yes

See Appendix 4 for a list of emotions.

Is This The Root?

Sometimes it is good to ask this question. Consider the word 'love'. There are at least 20 words for which love is the root – 21 with the word 'love' itself. In case you do not believe me, here they are:

- Beloved
- Lovably
- Loveable
- Love
- Loved
- Loveless
- Loveliness
- Lovelorn
- Lovely
- Lovesick
- Lovemaking
- Lover
- Lovers
- Lovey
- Loving
- Lovingly
- Unlovable
- Unloved
- Unlovely
- Unloving
- Unlovingly

You could ask the question 'Is the word love', get the answer 'no' and go off in a completely different direction. To avoid this a questioning sequence might look like this:

- Is love the root of this word? Yes
- Is it love? No
- Is it an adjective? Yes
- Is it an 'un' word? Yes
- Is it unlovable? No
- Unloved? Yes

Useful Books

Reference books can be very useful in helping you find that illusive word. In general, dictionaries are not a lot of help because they only list synonyms. A thesaurus is much more useful. The term Roget's Thesaurus is not a guarantee of quality as the term is now out of copyright so anyone can publish a Roget's Thesaurus. My favourite is sadly out of print: *Roget's International Thesaurus* edited by Robert L Chapman, published by Collins in the UK and Harper Collins in the USA. If you do a lot of "word work" I suggest you get a second-hand copy of this, but do make sure it is edited by Robert L Chapman. In my opinion it is by far the best Roget's Thesaurus you will find. Try www.abebooks.com. When I looked they had lots of these available very cheaply second hand.

The other book I recommend is *Collins Concise Thesaurus*. This is very simple to use, and includes antonyms (opposites) as well as synonyms. It lacks the depth of the other book, but will often be a great help.

PLACEMENT: WHERE IS IT?

Sometimes you need to place something on the body as part of a procedure, or an activity needs to be done in a particular place, or sometimes you are trying to locate something that is needed for a particular procedure.

Scanning & Putting Things On The Body

Sometimes a client needs to wear something (e.g. a crystal), or something has to be placed on the body as part of an energy procedure (e.g. a magnet, a crystal or coloured light), so systematic questioning is often required to identify the exact spot quickly. Occasionally it does not matter where the object is placed, as long as it is on the body, so a preliminary question is often in order, such as:

- Is it important where the crystal is placed?

Assuming you get 'yes' to this, you then need to ask some more questions. I have found that the best way is to view the body as a box (with a front, back, two sides, a top and a bottom). I do not tell this to the client, because it sometimes brings coffins to mind!

If you establish that it is on the front of the body, you would then ask further questions, such as:

- Is it above the navel? (I choose the navel rather than the waist, because on some people the waist is an extremely imprecise place!)

or

- Is it placed on the legs?

I usually establish a general area in this way, and then use scanning to establish the exact spot. A light continual pressure is used while scanning along a line just off the body, using a finger or a pointer. When the muscle gives way, you are at the required point on the line.

So, for example, if the object is going to be on the front of the body above the navel, I scan from the neck to the navel on the mid-line asking for the arm to go down when I get to the correct level. I then ask if I need to go towards me or away from me. When I have established this, I scan in that direction again looking for the arm to go down when I get to the correct spot.

John Payne, my partner, feels that asking the arm to go down is contrived and inconsistent, and unnecessary. He finds the general area as before, then points to roughly the mid-point of that area and asks:

- Does the point lie above here?

If he get 'yes' he then scans upwards from that spot asking repeatedly:

- Is it above here?

Once again the arm will go down when he gets to the right spot.

The reasons for using a system where you are looking for an unlocked response only when you get to the right spot is that repeated unlocking of the muscle is both tiring for the client and slows the testing as you have to keep resetting the arm in the test position.

Whichever method I use, I finally I ask two check questions:

- Is this in exactly the correct place?
- Do I need to change this in any way?

While you are doing the scanning do not hold the object in your hand, as this can distort the results because the body can become unbalanced.

Scanning can also be used to find an item on a list or in a box.

Locating A Particular Place

When locating a particular place, you need to first find the general area. This may be clear from the context of the questioning. The place may be very specific (e.g. the client's bedroom, a particular beauty spot, etc.) or more general (e.g. anywhere as long as it is outdoors, by the ocean, in a small dark room, etc.). This needs to be determined first by questions such as:

- Is this a specific place?
- Is this a general place that has specific characteristics?

Once this is established, the exact location can be narrowed down. If the location is a specific place, these sort of questions would be appropriate:

- Is this a specific place known to the client?
- Do I (the practitioner) have experience of this place?
- Is this inside a building?

If it is a general place that has specific characteristics, you will need to ask a different series of questions, e.g.

- Is the place we are looking for outdoors?
- Is this a place the client would find pleasant?
- Is the level of light or noise important?
- Is it important whether or not other people are there?

Locating An Object

Sometimes it is useful to find an object needed during or after the session by finding its location. You could be looking for a unique object (e.g. the client's lipstick, a particular crystal, the toilet cleaner in your toilet), or you could be looking for one of many examples of this that you could locate easily (e.g. a mirror, anything as long as it is a particular shade of red, something furry, something icy cold, etc.). So first you need to establish whether it is a totally unique object. Although a client's lipstick is not totally unique, because there will be more in the store, for the purposes of this it would be classified as unique, as it is the only one available. Questioning might look like this:

- Are we looking for a unique object? Yes
- Does it belong to you? Yes
- Do you have this with you at the moment? Yes
- Is it in your bag? No
- Is it in the pocket of your coat? Yes (client empties pocket)
- Is it this? Yes

ESTABLISHING QUANTITIES: HOW MUCH?

There are various situations in which you might want to establish how much of something is needed. For example, finding the optimum amount of fresh vegetables to enhance health, or the maximum amount of something that a person can tolerate without experiencing a reaction or without damaging their health. Establishing this sort of information can take a long time if it is not done systematically.

How Are We Going To Measure?

The important thing with this sort of testing is that you give the client instructions that they can use in practice. This is easy for things like supplements as this is usually expressed as a number of tablets / capsules. Things get more complicated when we want to measure food and drink.

The usual options for foods are:

- Ounces
- Grams
- Spoonfuls (e.g. teaspoons, table spoons)
- Cups (particularly for American and Canadians)
- Standard portions
- Units (e.g. slices of bread, number of grapes, etc.)
- Percentage terms

The usual options for liquids are:

- Fluid ounces
- Pints
- Millilitres

- Cups/glasses
- Units (e.g. whisky measures, bottles of beer, etc.)
- Percentage terms

Give the client various options and ask if they have a preference, e.g. would they prefer ounces, grams or spoonfuls? If they would prefer spoonfuls, ask them what size spoon would they prefer etc. For some things you might want to use the measure 'normal portion' or 'typical slice of bread' or 'my favourite mug'. If you are doing this, ask the client to indicate with their hands how big this is before you start doing the questioning. For extra reliability you can also ask the client to imagine the measure as you do the testing.

For some things you also need to ask the client if they want you to express the amount as total quantity or as additional quantity. For example, if you are checking water intake for a client, you could express it in terms of total amount (e.g. eight glasses a day), or in terms of the amount additional to their current intake (e.g. three glasses a day).

How Much?

Before you ask any of these questions be clear in your own mind if you are asking minimum, maximum or optimum.

- Minimum: if people are short of money or reluctant to do something, you might want to ask for the minimum for the person to receive any benefit.
- Maximum: if you are looking at something that is basically not good for the person, you may want to know what is the maximum they can have / do without experiencing a problem. When you get the result to this, it is important that you explain to the client that the body is not saying they must drink three cups of coffee a day, for instance, but is saying this is the maximum that can be tolerated without harm.

- Optimum: this is for beneficial things where you are finding what will give the most benefit either in general or for a particular problem.

For example, the questioning might look something like this for establishing wheat quantity for a client with tolerance problems:
- What is the maximum amount of bread you should eat in a day if this is your only source of wheat – at least 5 slices? Yes (Client has previously used her hands to show me what a normal slice of bread looks like.)
- At least 5 slices? No
- Is it 3 slices? No
- Is it 4 slices? Yes
- If you have your favourite breakfast cereal, what is the maximum amount of bread – at least 2 slices? Yes
- At least 3 slices? Yes
- Is it a maximum of 3 slices? Yes
- If you have a normal portion of pasta and the breakfast cereal, what is the maximum amount of bread you should eat – 2 slices? Yes

I would probably leave it like this rather than work out all the possible combinations of bread / pasta / cereals / biscuits / cakes. I would summarise the information: you should have a maximum of four slices of bread a day, but, if you eat your favourite breakfast cereal, you should only have three slices of bread that day. If you also have pasta, only two slices of bread. I would then explain that if she ate biscuits or something similar she would need to adjust these figures, and also remind her of all the things she might eat that contain small amounts of wheat and would further reduce the permitted intake of bread.

So far we have just focussed on the wheat element in the bread, but it may be that she needs to restrict her intake of bread for some other reason. For example, she may be allergic / intolerant of the baker's yeast found in bread, or she may have problems with the butter she always puts on the bread (too much saturated fat / too many calories / allergy / intolerance), etc. This could mean that although five slices of bread is the correct maximum for the wheat, three is the maximum for the brewer's yeast, butter, or whatever. It is possible to build this into your initial questioning. This speeds things up, but can complicate things too. I keep changing my mind about which is the best approach, so I suggest you try both and decide for yourself.

If you wanted to include these other considerations in the initial question, you would phrase the question something like this:

- What is the maximum amount of bread you should eat in a day if this is your only source of wheat, and bearing in mind any other restricting factors – at least 3 slices?

In this example if the bread needs to be restricted because of baker's yeast, you might get three slices as the maximum (rather than the four when considering wheat alone). If you then add in the breakfast cereal, you would still get three slices, as the breakfast cereal does not contain any bakers yeast. This can seem very confusing, so you may prefer to ask the questions as I did initially and then ask some more questions such as:

- Are there any reasons you need to restrict your intake of bread, breakfast cereal or pasta further? Yes
- Is it the bread you need to restrict further? Yes
- So what is the maximum bread you should eat in a day – is it 3 slices? Yes
- Is this because of the baker's yeast in it? Yes
- Do you need to restrict your intake of other foods with yeast? Yes (discuss what other foods the client eats and test for these)
- Do you need to restrict the cereal or pasta further? No
- Is there anything else we need to know about this?

ESTABLISHING QUANTITIES: HOW MANY?

There are various times you might want to establish a number: finding the number of times a client needs to repeat an affirmation, establishing the correct number of times to take a flower remedy each day, finding the number of different things the client needs to think about, working out how many vials are needed from a test kit, or finding the right number of capsules to take, etc.

Establishing An Exact Number

There are several different ways of phrasing this sort of question. The fastest way to establish the exact number is to ask in one of the following ways:

- At least X: if you ask *Is it at least 4?* and get the answer "yes", then the number is 4, 5, 6 , 7, etc.
- X or more: this is the same as "at least X".
- More than X: if you ask *Is it more than 4?* and get the answer "yes" , then the number is <u>not</u> 4 , but would be 5,6,7,etc.
- Less than X: if you ask *Is it less than 4?* and get the answer "yes", then the number is 0,1,2 or 3.

Whichever method you use, choose a number to start with, and then according to the answer you usually ask about another number several higher or lower than the first number. The number you first start with depends on the circumstances, e.g. if you were checking the number of vitamin C tablets for the person to take you would probably start with, say, two, whereas if you were asking about the number of repetitions for a weight lifting routine for an experienced body builder you might want to start with fifteen or twenty.

Choose <u>one</u> of these methods and stick to it initially until you gain some experience and confidence. The first way is probably the most popular method, so this is the method used in the following example, where I want to establish the number of repetitions for a particular exercise for a body builder:

- Do you need to do at least 15 repetitions of this exercise? Yes
- At least 20? Yes
- At least 25? No (these last two questions tell you it has to be 20, 21, 22, 23 or 24)
- At least 22? No (this has now narrowed it down to 20 or 21)
- Is it 20? No
- Is it 21? Yes
- So, you need to do 21 repetitions of this exercise, is that correct? Yes

TIME: HOW OFTEN? WHEN?

How Often? When?

We may want to know how often a person needs to do something. For example we may want to establish how often someone takes a supplement, or when they need to take a flower remedy, etc.

I used to assume that whenever I was working in this area I would be working according to clock time or calendar time, e.g. at 6.30 p.m., three times a day, every other day, etc. Then one day I was working with a client and had a lot of difficulty establishing when she needed to do something. After a lot of head scratching I realised that there was the possibility of activity time, so that something is done at the same time as another activity. So now whenever I am faced with a time question, I first ask:

- Are we measuring in clock time?

If I get 'no' to this, I ask:

- Are we measuring in activity time?

Clock Time (Also Known As Calendar Time)

This relates to a particular time of the day or repetitions expressed in terms of hours / days / weeks / months. So, for example:

- You need to take the supplement 3 times per day.
- You need to go to the gym twice a week.
- You need to eat your breakfast before 8.00 a.m.
- You need to take these flower remedies every 3 hours.

If I am using clock time, I first want to find out which units I am working in:

- A precise time. (e.g. at 9.30 p.m., before noon)
- A precise interval of time. (e.g. every 2 hours)
- A precise number of times a day / week. (e.g. 3 times a day, twice a day)

It is often clear from the context which to use. If it is not, I ask a question like this:

- Am I looking for a precise time?

A questioning sequence for working out an exercise regime where you have already established through muscle testing that the client needs to go to the gym (a one hour session following the routine the gym instructor worked out six months ago) and also go swimming (fifteen hundred metres, medium pace, front crawl) might look like this:

- Do you need to go to the gym at least twice a week? Yes
- At least four times a week? No
- Twice a week? Yes
- Is there anything else we need to know about the gym? No
- For the swimming, is it at least three times a week? No
- At least twice a week? Yes
- So, it's twice a week? Yes
- Do we need to know anything else about the swimming? Yes
- Is it about the days it happens? Yes
- Do you need to swim on specific days of the week? No
- Is it in relation to the gym? Yes
- So, is it that you should swim on different days to going to the gym? Yes
- Is there anything else we need to know about the swimming? No

Activity Time

These relate to a particular activity. So, for example:

- You need to take two of your supplements with your breakfast and one with your evening meal.
- You need to avoid eating wheat when you eats oranges.
- You need to do a series of stretching exercises immediately after you go for a run.
- You need to eat breakfast before getting dressed but after doing your visualisation.
- You need to sleep for an extra hour on days that you see more than six clients. If you see more than eight clients, you also need to take some specific flower remedies.
- You need to increase your zinc supplement in the week before your period.
- You must avoid all alcohol while you are pregnant.
- You need to avoid all dairy on days when you do not rest for at least fifteen minutes in the afternoon.

The main options are:

- Before the activity (e.g. before eating breakfast).
- At the same time as the activity (e.g. whenever milk is drunk).
- After the activity (e.g. after exercise).
- When the activity does not happen (e.g. when the client does not chew their food slowly).

A questioning sequence, where you have established that the client needs to say an affirmation, might look like this:

- Is it important when the affirmation is said? Yes
- Are we looking for clock time? No
- Activity time? Yes
- Is it before a particular activity? Yes
- Is this activity something that you normally find stressful? Yes (the fact that this is an affirmation suggests this as a strong possibility.)

- Is it done before anything you find stressful? No (conversation with client about what she finds stressful – visiting her mother, going to the supermarket, speaking out at meetings at work, doing her tax return.)
- Is it any of these? Yes
- Is it visiting your mother? Yes
- Do we need to know anything more about this? Yes
- Do we need to be more precise about the time before? Yes
- Is it as you drive over? No
- Once you've stopped the car at your mother's house? Yes
- So, you need to say your affirmation in the car once you've stopped outside your mother's house. Is that correct? Yes
- Anything else we need to know about this? No
- Any other times you need to do the affirmation? Yes
- One or more of the other times you've mentioned as being stressful? Yes
- etc.

TIME: HOW LONG?

How Long?

We often want to know how long a person needs to continue
something. For example, how many days or weeks or months to
take a supplement, how long to avoid wheat, how long an exercise
regime should be carried out for before a re-check, etc.

Once again there are the two possibilities of clock time, e.g.

- Until 16th February.
- Until 5.00 p.m.
- Until Thursday.
- Indefinitely.

and activity time, e.g.

- Until the next appointment.
- Until you stop taking the contraceptive pill.
- As long as you do this job.
- As long as you smoke.

Clock Time

You can work in days, weeks, etc., but you still then have to
convert that into an actual date, so in general I work with dates.

One possibility is that the client needs to do something indefinitely.
In practice I feel it is important to test this again in a maximum of
six months, because unforeseen things can happen.

A questioning sequence might look like this:

- Do we work in clock time? Yes
- Is this indefinitely? No
- Is this at least until the end of this month (January)? Yes
- At least until the end of February? No
- At least until 15th February? Yes
- At least until 20th February? No
- At least until 18th February? No
- Till 15th February? No
- Till 16th February? Yes
- Is this accurate enough? Yes

For some things you need to be even more precise. I find this often happens when testing has shown that a person needs to wear a magnet for a while. The time to remove the magnet is often very precise, e.g. 4.30 p.m. on 19th January.

Activity Time

When activity time is involved, there are two different options:

- Until some activity stops.
- Until some activity starts.

The most common activity time is until the next appointment, so I would normally ask about this first. A questioning sequence where you have already established that the client needs to drink four extra glasses of water a day, but need to know for how long, might look like this:

- Are we going to use activity time? Yes
- Is it until the next appointment? No
- Is it until some activity stops? Yes
- Is it some activity you have been considering stopping? No (client has previously told me that he was thinking of giving up smoking and going on a diet)

- Is it something that you know is bad for him? Yes (consultation with client, who admits he drinks a lot of beer and wine, regularly eats junk food often late at night)
- Is it one of the things we have just discussed? Yes
- Is it the beer and / or wine? No
- Is it the junk food? Yes
- Is this regardless of when the junk food is eaten? Yes
- So as long as you eat junk food regularly you need to drink 4 extra glasses of water a day. Is that correct? Yes

What Happens Then?

It is important not to assume that when the time is over that the activity stops. The activity could:

- Increase (e.g. more repetitions of an exercise or more frequent gym visits).
- Reduce (e.g. take 2 capsules instead of 3).
- Stop.
- Change in some way (e.g. supplement now taken at a different time of the day)
- Alternate (e.g. take a different type of calcium for three weeks, then back to the original one for four weeks and so on).

If the activity is continuing till the next appointment, you can check out during that appointment what should happen next. If the person is not coming back for another appointment, or the appointment date is after the final date for the activity, you need to check at the time what happens after this date:

- Do you then stop the activity?

ALLERGY & INTOLERANCE TESTING

General Questions

People can be allergic literally to anything, so do not exclude anything from your testing. You need your verbal questioning skills to narrow down the possibilities. First check how many different allergens or components you are looking for. You can review how to do this under the section 'Establishing Quantity: How Many?'

You then use further questions to narrow down the area, e.g.
- Is it a food?
- Is it something drunk?
- Is it personal care products? (e.g. shampoo, deodorant, toothpaste, cosmetics, etc.)
- Is it household products?(e.g. washing powders, bathroom cleaners, etc.)
- Is it something the person inhales? (e.g. house dust mite, pollens, perfume, etc.)
- Is it something the person touches?(e.g. metal, fabric, wood, etc.)
- Is it something the person takes? (e.g. nutritional supplement, drugs, etc.)
- Is it something taken in accidentally? (e.g. plastic sucked on a pen, remains of washing up liquid on cutlery, etc.)
- Is it something specifically to do with the person's work?

Do remember that all allergens are not necessarily from the same category, e.g. your client could be allergic to her perfume, nickel and bananas.

Which Food Is It?

People are often allergic to foods that they particularly like, so it is always worth asking the question:

- Are we looking for a favourite food?

If you get the answer 'yes', ask the client about their favourite foods and then test each of these in turn. If none of these show up, ask them to give you the names of more favourite foods. If this does not produce a result, you will need to be more systematic.

I use two ways of categorising foods to narrow down the options:

- Culinary categories (e.g. meat, fish, cakes and pastries, etc.)
- Botanical categories (e.g. lily family, deadly nightshade family, etc.)

To find out more about these categories see appendix 3. Note that these are different ways of classifying the same things, so all simple foods appear in both categories. For example, you could find carrot via culinary category (vegetables) and via botanical categories (parsley family). So when you are asking the question, you are asking for the easiest way to find the food. The botanical list is particularly useful for some of the less obvious things. The culinary categories are often useful for finding more complex foods (e.g. the burger the client eats from time to time). So the questioning might look like this:

- Is the easiest way to find this food using culinary categories? No
- Is it using botanical categories? Yes
- Is it on the first page of my list? No
- Is it on the second page of my list? Yes
- etc.

Another way of narrowing down the options is to ask when the client commonly eats the food, e.g.

- Is the food we are looking for normally eaten at most meals? No
- Is the food eaten at one or more specific meals? No
- Is it usually eaten between meals? Yes (consult client on sort of things eaten between meals)
- Is it biscuits? No
- Is it chocolate? No (consult client again, who then remembers that has a packet of chewing gum that she keeps in the car and chews while driving)
- Is it the chewing gum? Yes
- Is it all chewing gum? Yes

Avoiding Or Reducing Intake

Sometimes a client will need to avoid the substance completely, either indefinitely or for a period of time, but sometimes they will need to reduce their intake. If they need to reduce their intake, you need to find out for how long.

Some years ago I had a client who was severely allergic to fish: his throat would begin to close up with even the smallest amount of fish stock. I carried out various energy procedures to correct this, but testing then showed that it would take six months before he could eat any fish without reacting. I tested how much he could eat that first time and it was a very small quantity. I tested how long he must wait before he ate more fish and how much it should be. It took quite a while to work out an extremely detailed programme for his fish intake, but testing showed that he would eventually be able to eat several varieties of fish in normal quantities. Normally I do not work out such a detailed programme as this, but because of his severe and potentially life-threatening reaction to all fish, I felt it was imperative to do so. When I saw him again many months later, he told me that he had followed my instructions to the letter and was now eating fish without any problem.

Banking Food

When working with intolerance the concept of 'banking food' is useful. For example, you might work out that a client can tolerate twenty grams of chocolate a day, or a quarter of a cup of coffee a day. The client may well ask if it is possible to save this up and have it all at one time. I developed the concept of 'banking food' in response to this sort of question. I have found that the easiest way to phrase a question to answer this type of query from a client is to ask:

- How many days would it be appropriate for you bank food –at least three?

You ask this and similar questions till you find the exact number of days. For example, if you tested five for the coffee, you would explain to the client that they can have a quarter of a cup of coffee a day, or save it up and have half a cup every two days, or a full cup every four days, or a cup and a quarter every five days. They can vary what they do, but they can't 'save' the coffee for longer than five days or 'draw out' any more than what they have saved at any particular time.

Beneficial Food

As well as testing for food quantity where tolerance is a problem, you might also want to test for quantity of beneficial food (ones that enhance vital energy). Here you would be testing for the optimum to eat, rather than the maximum to avoid harm. Nevertheless the questioning is very similar, although banking food is not usually an issue.

When I am seeking to establish the category of food I usually use three categories (see appendix 3):

- Culinary categories (e.g. meat, fish, cakes and pastries, etc.)

- Botanical categories (e.g. lily family, deadly nightshade family, etc.)
- Nutritional categories (e.g. food containing zinc, polyunsaturated oils, etc.)

Confirmation

If you have a procedure for testing for allergy, intolerance and vital energy that does not involve asking verbal questions, it is good to use this to confirm what you have just found.

Read my books *Allergy A To Z* for more information on allergies, and *Nutritional Testing For Kinesiologists And Dowsers* for more information on nutritional testing.

NUTRITIONAL SUPPLEMENTS

Accuracy

The most accurate way of testing supplements is to have a supplement there while you ask the question. Many manufacturers now provide testing kits of their supplements, and these allow you to have access to a wide range of supplements without incurring a great deal of expense. Some branches of kinesiology teach that the supplement should be put on the client's body while the testing takes place. I generally like to have it in my hand or close by while testing verbal questions.

If the client brings an unfamiliar supplement in for testing, I normally read what it says on the label, take a capsule out, look at it and smell it before starting the questioning.

There are occasions when you want to do some questioning but do not have a supplement available. In general you will get more accurate answers if you and / or the client have experience of the supplement. Testing off lists when neither you nor the client has any experience of the supplement is likely to be the least accurate.

What Are You Testing For?

You need to be clear in your mind before you start supplement testing what standard you are testing to:

- Supplements needed to avoid gross deficiency signs.
- Supplements to maintain or improve general health and well-being.
- Supplements for a particular problem.

Two Different Situations

There are two main possibilities:

- The person may already be taking supplements and you want to check if everything is correct.
- The person may not be taking any supplements at all.

The procedure I recommend is slightly different depending on which of these situations you have.

Client Already Taking Supplements

First look at the existing supplements that are being taken. There are five basic possibilities for each supplement:

- It is beneficial and optimal.
- It is beneficial but not the best one to take (e.g. client does need a multi-vitamin supplement but not the one they are currently taking)
- It is beneficial, and the best source, but something about it needs to be changed (dose, time taken, avoid / have at same time, etc.).
- It is harmful.
- It is having no effect.

For each supplement ask which of these categories applies. If the second option, you need to find an alternative either from the same manufacturer or from an alternative manufacturer. If the third option, work out what needs changing, e.g.

- Is this vitamin C supplement beneficial and optimal? No
- Beneficial but not best source? No
- Beneficial but something needs to be changed? Yes
- Is the dose correct? Yes
- Is the time that it's taken correct? No (client takes in the morning on an empty stomach)

- Should the vitamin C supplement be taken with food? Yes
- Do we need to know anything else about the vitamin C supplement? Yes
- At a particular meal? Yes
- Breakfast? Yes
- So the vitamin C supplement should be taken with breakfast? Is that correct?
- Anything else we need to know about the vitamin C supplement? No

When you have checked each supplement the client is currently taking, ask if any others need to be added, and if so follow the same procedure as for clients who are not taking anything to find the additional supplements.

Client Not Taking Any Supplements At The Moment

Check first of all that the client needs to take supplements.

It is possible to work out the supplements in two different ways:

- Finding the type of nutrient first e.g. 500 mg of vitamin C and then finding a supplement that matches this.
- Finding the supplement that is best.

In general the second approach is the easiest, e.g.

- Do I have a sample of this supplement here? Yes
- Is it one of brand X? No
- Is it one of brand Y? Yes
- etc.

If it is a supplement that you do not have there, you can ask if it is one that you know about or the client knows about.

Once you have found the supplement, you need to check what the dose is and how it should be taken. Normally I first look at the standard does that is recommended by the manufacturer, and I ask:

- Do you take the supplement as detailed on the packet? Yes

I would then ask:

- Is there anything else we need to know about this supplement?

Because it could be that there is some additional instruction that is necessary. For example, the manufacturer's instruction might say that the standard dose is one tablet a day with food, but the full instruction for the client could be one tablet a day with food, and the client should also eat some vitamin C rich food at the same time to enhance absorption.

If the client does not take the supplement as indicated on the packet, you would need to work out all the details of dose and timing, e.g.

- Do you take at least two tablets a day? Yes
- More than two? No
- Are both tablets taken at the same time? No
- Is one or both taken with meals? Yes
- Etc.

Read my book *Nutritional Testing For Kinesiologists And Dowsers* for more information on nutritional testing.

TESTING FOR REMEDIES
& TEST KIT VIALS

There are many occasions when you might want to test for flower
or gem remedies, work out which homeopathic remedy would be
best to take, or find a test kit vial to use as part of an energy
procedure. The testing is similar in many ways to testing for
nutritional supplements, so look again at that section.

Accuracy

As with supplements you are likely to do your most accurate testing
if you have the remedies or vials there. Testing off a list will work
if you are very familiar with what you are testing.

Narrowing Down The Type

You may have several different types of flower remedies, or several
different test kits, so you need first to narrow down the options, by
establishing which it is, e.g.

- Am I looking for a Bach Flower Remedy? No
- Am I looking for an Australian Bush Remedy? Yes

Or

- Am I looking for something out of the bacteria test kit? No
- Out of the virus test kit? No
- Out of the fungus test kit? No
- Out of one of the parasite test kits? No
- Out of the hormone test kit? Yes

Finding The Exact Remedy Or Vial

Having established the kit or box it is in, you next need to narrow it down to the specific one. Some practitioners place the remedies on the client's body while they ask questions. I prefer to have the box or kit next to me. If the vials are in a box, I run my finger along a row of them and ask:

- Is it one of these?

If I get 'yes', I ask about half of the row and so on until I pin down the exact bottle or vial.

If the vials are in a bag, I take out a small handful and ask about that, using the same question as when the vials are in a box.

Confirmation

If you have a procedure for testing for remedies that does not involve asking verbal questions, it is good to use this to confirm what you have just found.

INDEXES

Indexes (or indices) can be extremely useful; they can also give a spurious scientific appearance to the work we do, so they need to be used with care. They can be used in many different situations to give you and the client additional information. Judicious use of indexes can help you to work more effectively and can help clients to make more informed decisions.

One of the problems with kinesiology is that you will always get an answer to your question, but you do not know for certain that this is an accurate answer. Working with indexes can be particularly fraught in this way. When I first started to use indexes I used them for testing improvements. I did it silently, made a note of the result and then monitored what happened to the client. With time I became convinced that I could generally be accurate.

In a book like this I can only give some indications of the way in which indexes can be used. I suggest you work with them in the ways discussed here to develop your skills in this area, but with time you will see many other possible applications.

Numerical Indexes

These are the ones that are most commonly used – scales chosen are usually 0 to 10 or 0 to 100. The scale 0 to 100 suggests an extreme level of precision – that you can accurately detect through muscle testing a difference between an index of 56 and one of 57. If you recognise that you cannot do this, use a scale of 0 to 10, or else test across ranges, e.g.

- Is it between 55 and 60?

You stop at this level, if the answer is "yes". Only proceed to a more exact number if you are certain that the difference is meaningful.

Calibrating The Scale

Do not proceed with muscle testing until you have defined what you mean by 0 and what you mean by 10 (or 100). It is not enough to say best and worse. What do you mean by this? For example, I define a geopathic stress level of 100 as being a place where people would die instantly because of the geopathic stress problems.

Sometimes I check out organ function. O is fairly easy to define (no discernable activity or output from the organ, or the organ is absent). 100 can be defined in several different ways, and I use different definitions depending on circumstances:

- 100 = the perfect organ function.
- 100 = the best possible function for that person.
- 100 = the best that the organ can function with the knowledge and expertise that I as a practitioner have.
- 100 = the best function that organ has ever had in that person's life so far.

Comparing Things Using Indexes

This is an extremely useful way of using indexes. I usually arbitrarily allocate a score of 100 to one of the items / actions, and then compare others with it. If the score for the second item is more than 100, it is better for that person, and if the score is less than 100, it is worse. Alternatively, you could test for an exact figure for the starting item. This adds an extra complicating step, and is unnecessary if you really want just to focus on the relative merits of two or more things.

- 68 -

A typical situation when you might want to use this type of index is for comparing supplements or comparing different types of water. For example, the client has already bought a cheaper version of the supplement you are recommending. You arbitrarily allocate an index of 100 to the supplement the client has, and then index the recommended supplement against it. If the recommended supplement is 102, the client will probably decide to take what they have and then possibly buy the recommended one when the first one is finished. If the recommended supplement is 542, the client may decide immediately to buy the recommended supplement. This use of indexing gives the client valuable information on which to make decisions.

You could do a similar thing for looking at the impact of suggested changes on their health. This is particularly useful to do when clients are reluctant to make a health investment. Once again you arbitrarily allocate a 100 to their current health and then check the impact the recommended changes would have on the client's health. A questioning sequence might look like this:

- If 100 is your current overall health index, what would the index be if you followed the exercise programme we've just worked out – at least 110? Yes
- At least 120? No
- At least 115? Yes
- So it would increase it to somewhere between 115 and 120? Yes
- What would the index be if you just took the flower remedies as recommended – at least 110? Yes
- At least 115? No
- So somewhere between 110 and 115? Yes
- If you did both the exercise programme and the flower remedies what effect would that have on the index – at least 125? Yes
- More than 125? No
- So somewhere between 120 and 125? Yes

You could also check how long it would be before this benefit would be evident in the client's life.

Testing For Improvement

Indexes can be used to test for improvements. You test for an index for the current state of an organ, system, function, etc. and then test what it will be after the work has been completed. You can also re-test the index session by session. I have found that in general clients only notice a difference if an index increases by about twenty points, and this seems surprisingly to be independent of the starting point for the index. So, if the organ function is forty and by the next session it will be sixty five, the client is likely to be aware of some beneficial change, but if the score goes up to fifty five, they may well not be.

A client came to see me who had gone to her doctor feeling very unwell. Tests had shown her to be severely anaemic and also to have extremely low stores of iron. The doctor had prescribed iron tablets that morning, but she had not started taking them. Testing produced the following information:

- Her intake of iron currently compared with what should be: 65
- Her utilisation of iron currently compared with what should be: 11

If she took the iron supplement from her doctor:

- Intake of iron compared with what should be: 77
- Utilisation of iron compared with what should be: 11 (it is possible that if the form was particularly easy to assimilate, that utilisation would have increased too)

Her energy system asked for a whole range of procedures to be carried out, and did not want anything done at this point about increasing iron intake. Testing showed that when the work from that session was fully integrated, utilisation would increase dramatically to 53, and that another appointment needed to be scheduled for a month later. When the client returned for her second appointment, she told me she was feeling much better, and that she had taken the iron tablet from the doctor as we had agreed.

She had had another blood test, and the doctor was astounded at how much it had improved. This is not surprising, because he was unaware of the work that had been done by me on increasing her iron absorption and was just expecting to find an improvement as a result of increasing her iron consumption.

Nutritional Indexes

A score of 100 for an overall nutritional index would indicate that no improvement could be made in nutritional terms for that person. In practice this is highly unlikely to be achieved. It is relatively easy to get the index up into the eighties, but the remaining increase can be much more difficult to achieve. An index of 0 would mean it would not be possible to make it worse (although it may be possible to make it equally bad).

When working out an index for the current situation it is important to have a time scale in mind, e.g. an index for the last week may be different to an index for the last year. Longer time scales are particularly appropriate if the person's life style and eating patterns are erratic.

Both insufficiency and excess will decrease a nutritional index.

If the index is below 100 then there are four possibilities:

- Make changes to diet.
- Introduce and/or make changes to one or more supplements.
- Energy work to enhance absorption etc.
- Life style changes.

Sometimes rather than using a numerical index I use a descriptive index:

- Disastrous   = actively creates illness.

- Very poor   = stops a sick person getting well.
- Poor   = hampers recovery.
- Neutral   = no effect or benefits and problems cancel each other out.
- Good   = some deficiencies but generally O.K.
- Very good   = no deficiencies.
- Excellent   = supports vibrant health.

Sometimes it is useful to ask what the index would be if the person did / did not do a particular thing, e.g. if the person gave up smoking, followed a specific exercise plan, ate more slowly, etc.

Testing for the time in the person's life at which a dietary index was highest can be useful, but be aware that the diet which was suitable then may not be suitable now (although in general there will be many factors in common).

Above all remember that whenever you are working with indexes, you are testing for a given individual, and, unless you specify otherwise, you are testing for an index for the current time. Things may change for a variety of reasons, and this could then change the index.

MANAGING THE SESSION

One of the most important uses of verbal questioning is in managing the treatment session. Sometimes it is difficult to know where to start, or to know whether a particular reaction that the client is experiencing is part of the healing process, or a sign that something is wrong.

Energy Permission

Health kinesiology practitioners are taught to be scrupulous about asking for energy permission to start and end a session. Other kinesiologists also should consider this to be an important part of the way they work.

The client may be keen for you to work on them, but it may not be appropriate. You may have another client waiting, but it may be extremely important that you carry out one more procedure.

Starting A Session

The session should always start with asking for energy permission. The person's conscious mind has given permission, because they are still on the couch, but occasionally there is a good reason why energy work would not be appropriate, even though the client may not be consciously aware of this. You should not proceed unless energy permission is given.

To establish energy permission you ask:

- Do we have energy permission to work together now?

The answer to this is usually 'yes'. If the answer is 'no', the session should stop there. The most common reason for not getting energy permission is that the client has recently visited another type of therapist. For example, the client may have recently been given a homeopathic remedy or had a shiatsu treatment and sometimes, but not always, it is just not appropriate to introduce even more changes, however beneficial they are in principal.

If the answer is 'yes', you proceed to the second question:

- Is there any reason why we should not work together now?

Usually the answer to this is 'no'. If you get this answer, you can proceed with the energy work. Occasionally there is some temporary reason why the practitioner should not proceed, but this is fixable immediately. In this case, you will get 'yes' as the answer to this question.

The exact things needing attention are identified through muscle testing. Common ones include giving the client a drink of water, making the client more comfortable in some way or explaining in more detail exactly what is going to happen. So, common questions you might want to ask include:

- Is this something you need to do? (e.g. go to the toilet, drink some water, etc.)
- Is this something I (the therapist) need to do? (e.g. go to the toilet, drink some water, tell the client something, etc.)
- Do we need to change something about the room? (e.g. dim or switch off lights, move the couch, open / close windows or doors, ask someone to leave the room, etc.)

The questioning sequence might look like this:

- Is this something you need to do? Yes
- Is it go to the toilet? No
- Is it drink water? No
- Is it to put on more clothes? Yes

- Would a cardigan be sufficient? Yes (client puts on cardigan)
- Is there any reason not to work together now? No

A new client came to see me, and initially I did not obtain energy permission to work unless I agreed that there were certain areas we would not touch on. The client made no comment about this. When I saw his sister a few days later for her appointment, she told me that he had told her what had happened. His wife also told her that just before his appointment he was listing all the things he was not prepared to talk to me about.

On one occasion I got 'yes' in answer to the second question and through muscle testing we established that I had to do something myself. Before the client had arrived I had made some soup (my office is an annex of my house). Once I started the session with the client I began to fret that I had not turned the soup off before I started work. I had to go and check the cooker. This was a reasonable instruction because I was hardly likely to do my best work while wondering if my house was about to burn down!

So to summarise:

	Question	Answer	Action
Question 1	Do we have energy permission to work together now?	Yes	Go to Question 2
Question 1	Do we have energy permission to work together now?	No	No further action or schedule an appointment at another time
Question 2	Is there any reason why we should not work together now?	Yes	Ask subsidiary questions to establish what needs to be done then ask Question 2 again

Question 2	Is there any reason why we should not work together now?	No	Start the work

What Do I Do First / Next?

Over the years I have spoken to students and practitioners of many different branches of kinesiology, and a dilemma that many experience is of knowing what technique or procedure to undertake first. This is particularly true for kinesiologists who have an eclectic mix of techniques gathered from several different training programmes. Some find using finger modes works well, but others either do not have enough knowledge to use finger modes effectively or prefer not to do so. Health kinesiology practitioners use a menu of techniques and procedures which quickly allows them to home in on the priority. This system can be adapted by other kinesiologists. I suggest you group together the procedures of a particular branch of kinesiology, using sub-headings if needed. You can also include other therapies that you practice, referral to other practitioners that you trust, and things the client needs to do for themselves (e.g. taking more exercise, saying an affirmation regularly, etc.). Here is how it might look, but I have used numbers and letters rather than actual names:

Kinesiology A:
      Technique 1
      Technique 2
            Technique 2a
            Technique 2b
      Technique 3
Kinesiology B:
      Technique 1
            Technique 1a
            Technique 1b

Technique 2
    Technique 2a
    Technique 2b
    Technique 2c
Technique 3
Other therapy A
Other Therapy B
Refer To Another Practitioner
    Therapist 1
    Therapist 2
Self-Help
    Action 1
    Action 2
    Action 3

Questioning might then look like this:

- Is the priority thing to do from kinesiology A? No
- Is it from kinesiology B? Yes
- Is it technique 1? No
- Is it technique 2? Yes
- Is it 2a? No
- Is it 2b? No
- Is it 2c? Yes
- So, the priority thing to do is technique 2c from kinesiology B. Is that correct?

You then work out anything else you need to know in order to perform that technique.

In asking these questions it is vital that we are clear what we mean by the word 'priority'. There seem to be three basic usages:

- It's the most important thing to do for that person.
- It's the next thing to do.
- It's O.K. to do it next.

In general I use the term to mean it is the first or next thing to do. This may seem as though I am not aiming very high, but if we liken kinesiology to cooking then in making an omelette the priority thing to do is to get the eggs out, even though this isn't the most important bit of the process.

Once you have completed that technique, ask if you have energy permission to do more work. If you get 'yes', run the menu again from the beginning to find the next thing to do.

How Many Sessions Are Needed?

Prospective clients often ask: "How many sessions will I need?" There is no standard answer: it depends entirely on the individual. The number of sessions does not necessarily even relate to the severity of the problem, nor does it relate to the length of time that the client has had the symptoms. I have had clients with a small patch of eczema who have needed five or six sessions to see the benefit, and I have also had some truly miraculous results for severe or long-standing problems in the space of one or two sessions. It is possible, with experience, to test for this, e.g.

- How many sessions are needed – at least 2?

Normally I book clients in for an hour, but occasionally muscle testing will dictate things differently. I had a client with vertigo who needed six or seven ten-minute appointments, rather than one one-hour one. You have to be guided by the muscle testing and proceed at the correct pace for the individual client.

Working On Several Different Problems At The Same Time

In a simple world we would work on one symptom or illness at a time, but life and clients are not quite like that. Sometimes clients come in with many different problems. When you work in priority order, you may be doing work for several symptoms at the same time, and then change to another procedure and do work for some of the same symptoms but not all of them. Often you do not need to analyse this, because you can just trust that everything will work out in the end, but sometimes it helps you to keep track of what is supposed to be happening if you map it out. I developed 'grid analysis' to deal with this situation. You set out the client's symptoms / goals and the procedures you will be doing in a grid. I have given simple examples here – I usually only use this sort of analysis where I am dealing with a client with seven or more symptoms / issues. There are two examples. The first is an adapted version of the grid analysis I use in my practice, making it suitable for use by all kinesiologists. The second example is the way health kinesiology students and practitioners might use it if the work to be done is organised into a sequence of issues.

Here is a simplified grid analysis that any kinesiologist could use or adapt:

	Symptom A	Symptom B	Symptom C	Goal D
1st Appointment	X		X	X
Action 1	X			
Action 2	X Complete		X	
Action 3				
Action 4			X	
2nd Appointment				
Action 1			X	
Action 2			X	
Action 3			X	
Action 4				X
Action 5				X
Homework			X Complete	

You write in the names of the symptoms across the top, and then write the name of each procedure that you carry out in the left hand column.

What does this grid tell us? It tells us several things:

- By the time the client comes back for their second appointment you would expect to see a substantial improvement or the complete absence of symptom A (unless the work was still being integrated).
- You would not expect to see any improvement in symptom B after the first two sessions, because you have not worked on it yet.
- You would probably not see much improvement in symptom C and goal D after the first session.
- The homework after the second session will have an effect on symptom C only.
- Further sessions will be needed to complete the work on Goal D and to start the work on symptom B.
- Etc.

Here is an example of a simplified grid analysis suitable for health kinesiologists:

	Symptom A	Symptom B	Symptom C	Goal D
Issue 1	X		X Complete	
Issue 2	X			X
Issue 3	X			X
Issue 4	X Complete			X
Issue 5				X

This grid tells us:

- You would not expect to see any improvement in symptom B, because you have not worked on it within the first five issues.
- You would not see any movement for Goal D after completing issue 1, and even after completing issues 1-5 you will still have not done all the work necessary for Goal D.

- Symptom C is completed after completing issue 1.
- Etc.

I do not use grid analysis very often, because it is time consuming, but complex clients with complex problems really appreciate the clarity this can bring to the sessions.

Scheduling The Next Appointment

Sometimes you do not need specifically to ask whether there is further work to do, because it has become clear earlier in the session that a programme of work is necessary, which will take more than a single session. Sometimes it is not clear, or a body of work has been completed, but you may wonder if there is more energy work needed in another area. On these occasions you need to ask:

- Is there any more work to schedule?

If there is more work, it is important to know when the next appointment should be scheduled. There are various ways of asking this, but a typical question would be:

- When should our next session be – on or before X?

I used to use number of days or weeks, but then I had to calculate what that meant in terms of an actual date, so I switched to asking about actual calendar dates. A question session might look like this:

- Is there any more work to schedule? Yes
- Is it before the end of the month (February)? No
- Is it before the end of March? Yes
- Is it on or before the 15th March? No
- Is it on or before the 25th March? Yes
- Is it on or before the 20th March? Yes
- Is it on or before 18th March? No
- Is it 19th March? No

- Is it 20th March? Yes
- So, the 20th March is the earliest date we should do more work. Is that correct?

Sometimes there is a time window. In other words the next lot of work must be completed within a certain time period. So to establish if this is necessary we need to ask this question:

- Is there an upper time limit?

If you get 'no' to this, you know that the work can be carried out on 20th March or any time after that without compromising what is being done. Obviously, in terms of getting better as soon as possible, it makes sense for the next appointment to be as close to 20th March as possible. If you got 'yes' to this question, you would then continue, e.g.

- Does the next appointment have to be done on 20th March? No
- Must it occur before the end of March? No
- Must it be before the end of April? No
- Before the end of May? Yes
- Is that precise enough? No
- So, before 15th May? Yes
- Before 10th May? Yes
- Before 5th May? No
- Before 8th May? Yes
- 5th May? Yes
- So the next session should be between 20th March and 5th May, including both those dates. Is that correct?

It is important to adhere to these time windows when they occur. A good example of this was some work I undertook on my partner, John Payne. When I met him, he had recurring bouts of illness characterized by sudden high temperatures and total prostration. This situation would occur every few months and last for several days. Testing showed that John was suffering from a recurring viral infection and that the virus would 'hide' in his body between the attacks. The work of the first session was to bring the virus into the blood stream so that it could be worked on. The energy system indicated that once this work had been done, it would take some time before the virus was in the blood stream. In fact, the body was extremely precise: the next session had to take place between 20th and 24th December. Testing subsequently showed that the virus would be 'available' in the blood stream by 20th December, so this explained the start date for the time window. The completion date for the time window was because, if the work were not done during that time, John would start to feel unwell and have another bout of the illness.

Information For The Next Session

Sometimes specific information about a session is needed ahead of time, and this can be gathered during a previous session by asking:

- Is there anything we need to know about the next session?

If you get, 'yes' to this, there are several broad possibilities:

- The client may need to bring something. (e.g. the nutritional supplements they are currently taking so they can be tested, a plan of their house so it can be checked for geopathic stress problems, the hair of their pet cat for allergy testing, etc.)
- The client may need to be told about the reaction they will have to the next session. (e.g. they may need to be aware that they are going to going to feel unwell temporarily immediately after the appointment so it would be advisable to bring someone with them to drive them home, or they may be going to feel extremely tired for a few days after the next appointment so should schedule an easy few days after that appointment, etc.)

This sort of information can be found by asking this sort of question:

- Does the client need to bring something?
- Does the client need to know something now about their reaction to the next session?

If the answer is 'yes' to either of these questions, further questioning is needed.

What Will Be The Benefit Of The Work We've Done?

It is possible to ask this question simply in relation to the problem that you are addressing in the session, or you can open the question up: because kinesiology is such a holistic therapy clients will often notice improvements in symptoms that you are not even aware of. I will always remember the client who said as he was leaving: "By the way, that pain's gone." He had never told me about a pain, so I was puzzled. He then explained that he had had a pain in his side for over twenty years. Hospital investigations had never shown anything significant, but now, in the middle of his treatment for an apparently unrelated problem, it had gone. Clients will quite frequently not tell you about some symptoms. There can be several reasons for this. For example, they may not want to sound like a hypochondriac; they may believe that nothing can be done about it, or they may feel it is normal for someone of their age to have these problems.

In practice I usually only ask about improvements in the client's presenting symptoms. I first ask a general question:

- Will David notice any significant benefit for any of his problems before the next session?

Sometimes there will not be any noticeable benefit from the work that has been done; the work may be laying foundations for what will happen in subsequent sessions. When asking this sort of question you are interested in asking about the client noticing the benefit, so I usually use their name in the questioning rather than 'you' to emphasise my intent. Not everyone is equally perceptive about themselves and their bodies. For example, I have had clients with eczema who seem unable to see that there has been an improvement until all their eczema has gone. When asking this question, I am clear in my intent that I am asking about David's perception not what mine would be in a similar situation.

One client came back for the second session and said triumphantly to me: "You were right. I am no better." The beginning of the second session could have been quite different if I had not asked the question in the previous session. In all likelihood the client would have cancelled his appointment or come back and complained that he had not experienced any improvement in his symptoms. Of course, you could test this at the beginning of the second session to establish that it is correct that the client has not experienced any improvement, but it is much less convincing for the client if it is done at this point.

I usually use the phrases 'significant benefit' or 'definite improvement'. By this I mean that the client will know that there is an improvement, and not be thinking: "Well, it seems a bit better" or something similar.

If you get 'yes' to the question at the end of the session, you probably will want to ask further questions to establish what that improvement might be. For example, for a client with eczema and sleep problems, where I have already established that there will be an improvement in both before the next session, I might ask various questions:

- Will the eczema cover less of your body?
- Will it be less red?
- Will it be less itchy?
- Will you find it easier to get to sleep?
- Will you wake less during the night?
- Will you wake later in the morning?
- Will you wake more refreshed?

I usually only focus on presenting symptoms, but sometimes it is appropriate to open the question up more widely. This is particularly true if the client needs to do something that is expensive, difficult or time-consuming. By finding all the benefits they will experience you can really motivate the client to embrace the necessary changes. I usually use the following categories to narrow down the improvements:

- Existing symptoms that the client has told me about, i.e. information I have listed on the client notes.
- Existing symptoms I do not know about.
- Physical body system (see appendix 1 for a list of these)
- Physical body part.
- Absorption / excretion of nutrients / toxins.
- Other body functions, e.g. easier breathing, greater ability to resist infection, etc.
- Weight (e.g. weight gain, weight loss, redistribution of fat).
- Other physical appearance improvements (e.g. glossier hair, stronger nails).
- Physical energy levels (e.g. overall increase, more stable energy levels, increase at a particular time of day / associated with an activity, etc.).
- Allergy / tolerance and addictive behaviour (e.g. able to eat more wheat without experiencing problems, easier to resist cigarettes, etc.)
- Strength / flexibility.
- Pain (e.g. less frequent, less severe, etc.)
- Sleep (e.g. easier to get to sleep, wake more refreshed, less disturbed during night, etc.)
- Sex (e.g. increased sexual libido, more satisfaction, increased sensitivity, easier / more reliable orgasms, etc.)
- Emotional symptoms (e.g. improvement in ability to control emotions in general or a specific emotion, higher levels of positive emotions in general or a specific emotion, fewer mood swings, greater self-confidence, higher self-esteem, etc.)
- Improved relationships (e.g. in general, with specific people or categories of people, etc.)

- Mental symptoms (e.g. improved memory, greater alertness, better concentration, etc.)
- Performance (e.g. improved performance in general, in work, in sport, etc.)
- Subtle energy (all corrections will affect subtle energy, but some may specifically affect a particular part of the subtle energy system e.g. integration of subtle bodies, balance of a chakra etc. Many people will be unaware of this sort of change, but a lot of therapists and energy-aware people will be).
- Spiritual (e.g. easier to engage in spiritual practice, heightened spiritual awareness, etc.)
- Preventive (although the client may well not be aware of this sort of benefit)
- Other

Having established that the client will indeed experience some improvement, this part of the questioning might look like this:

- Will Barbara be aware of any improvement in the symptoms she has told me about before the next session? Yes
- In her asthma? Yes
- Will she find it easier to breathe? Yes
- Anything else about the asthma? Yes
- Will she have fewer acute attacks? Yes
- Anything else about the asthma? No
- Will Barbara experience any improvement in any other of her symptoms she's told me about? No
- Will Barbara experience an improvement in symptoms she hasn't told me about? Yes. (I consult her about what other symptoms / problems she has, and she tells me she has arthritis and is worried about her memory.)
- Will she experience an improvement in one or both of these? Yes (If you got 'no' to this, you would need to prompt her for further symptoms)
- In both? No
- Just in the arthritis? No

- In the memory problems? Yes
- Any other improvements? Yes
- Etc.

Once you have some experience of this, it can be done very quickly.

What Will Happen If The Client Does Not Do Something?

As well as testing for the benefits of doing something, you can also test for what damage the client will do to themselves by not doing something. Questioning follows a similar line to the benefits questioning above, except you are focussing on the pains rather than the gains, e.g.

- If you don't give up smoking, will your health start to suffer? Yes
- Will any of your existing symptoms become worse? Yes
- Your headaches? Yes
- Any other of your symptoms? No
- Any thing else? Yes
- Will you start to experience respiratory symptoms? Yes
- Etc.

When Will The Improvement Be Noticeable?

Having established that the client will notice an improvement, the next obvious question is when. If the client is coming back for a follow-up appointment fairly quickly, I might not bother with this question, and just establish that the improvement will be experienced before the next session.

If this were the final appointment, I always test to find out when the client will experience the improvement. I usually check for two dates:

- When the client will experience a significant improvement.
- When the client will be symptom free, or as free as they are going to be as a result of the work we have done.

I then work out the two dates and write them down for them. I tell them to phone me if these do not transpire. Originally I only asked the second question, but I added the first question after an experience with a client who was in severe pain. I had told her she would be pain free in two months. She phoned me after two months and told me that she was still in as much pain as when she had left me after the last session. I asked her why she had waited till then to phone me, and she told me it was because I had given her the two-month time scale. When she came back in, I found I had made an error in her last session. If I had given her the first date as well (significant improvement), she would have contacted me sooner, and my error could have been rectified more quickly.

Once when I was telling a client to phone me if she did not experience the improvement I anticipated, I said: "If that doesn't happen, phone and moan." She laughed so much, I have used the phrase ever since.

Healing Process / Side Effects

Sometimes the client will feel worse either during the session or in the subsequent few days. This is common to many therapies and is usually referred to as a healing crisis, but Jimmy Scott, the founder of health kinesiology, prefers to refer to it as a healing process. He argues that the word 'crisis' implies something negative, whereas what is happening is something very positive.

It is possible to test for what uncomfortable reactions the client might have to the process. As the body goes through the healing process, the client might experience headaches, tiredness, unusual thirst, exacerbation of their existing symptoms, etc.

As the healing process can mean that the client appears to be worse after a session, it is important for you to be able to distinguish between a healthy healing process, and a treatment that has not worked. In general this is not difficult to do. If it is a healing process the client will, when questioned, often be able to identify some way in which the current situation is different from the normal symptoms. So, for example, the client might say that he normally loses his sense of smell when his sinuses are bad, but this time he has not, or that he is actually feeling cheerful and energetic, even though the pain is very bad. In addition, the healing process does not usually last longer than about five days.

At the end of a session you can test to see if a healing reaction is likely:

- Will you experience a healing reaction to this session?

Once again the question is specifically related to the client's perceptions, and you are making a projection not a prediction. If you get 'yes' to this question, you can find out what the healing process will involve, e.g.

- Will you experience unusual tiredness?

Energy Permission: Ending A Session

Deciding when to end a session is important, as the energy system may want a particular body of work completed in order to maximise results or minimise any uncomfortable effects of the healing process. Checking for energy permission to finish also protects the client against a mistake that you, the practitioner, might make.

Once again I use protocols based on health kinesiology. There are two basic questions:

- Do we have energy permission to stop?
- Is there any reason why we should not stop?

The first question gives a clear indication whether or not it is appropriate to stop now. If you get 'no' as an answer to this question, you need to find out what additional work you need to do. If you get 'yes', you ask the second question. These questions are vitally important because they help to safeguard the work that has been done. If the practitioner has omitted something important, the energy system will not give the practitioner permission to stop.

I had a very salutary experience of this some years ago. I had become rather lackadaisical about checking for energy permission to finish the session, and so sometimes I forgot this vital step. A client who had been making good progress phoned me up about three days after a treatment session. She told me that all the symptoms she had experienced in the last five years had come back. At the time I thought she was probably experiencing a healing process, so I asked her to leave it a few more days, and then phone me if she was still not well. Two days later she phoned me and told me that she could not stop crying, she had open weeping sores on her legs, her hands were blue all the time, and she had eight chilblains on her toes. I was alarmed by this and quickly booked her in for another appointment. When I looked at her notes, I realised that I had started by working out a whole body of work, but I had missed out one procedure when I actually came to do the work. I asked her energy system if it was appropriate just to do that particular procedure now, and it was. The procedure took about five minutes; as I worked I saw the colour slowly return to her hands. She was amazed by the speed of the transformation, and told me I was a miracle worker. I explained to her that, in fact, I had made an inexcusable mistake. If I had asked for energy permission to stop in the previous session, I am sure that I would not have been given it. The client had suffered six very uncomfortable days but was very philosophical about that. The outcome could have been much worse. Since that time I have been rigorous in asking for energy permission to stop a session.

Why Hasn't It Worked?

Sometimes clients return and say that nothing has changed, or even that they are worse. Careful questioning can often clarify what is going on. The actual questions depend on what happened during the previous session. One possibility is that you asked about improvement and got that there would be some. The other possibility is that you did not ask about what the benefit would be from the session. If you had not asked about improvement, the first question to ask is:

- Is everything going according to plan?

If you get the answer 'yes', you need to reassure the client and then continue on with the work. If you get the answer' no', you need to investigate. You also need to do this if you have tested for an improvement that has not occurred. There are several possibilities:

- Your testing about what would happen after the session was inaccurate.
- You did something wrong in the last session.
- Something has changed in the client's life that you could not have accounted for.

To establish which, I ask:

- Was I inaccurate in testing what would happen after the last session?

If I get 'yes' to this, I apologise to the client. I would still also check the other two options, because it is possible that I did more than one thing wrong, or the client also made some changes. So this is the question I now ask regardless of what answer I got to the first question:

- Did I do something wrong in the last session?

If I get 'yes' to this, there are two main possibilities:

- I missed something out.
- I did something wrong.

I would check both of these and then follow up on the 'yes'.

If I get 'yes' to the third question:

- Has something changed in your life?

I ask the client for suggestions and test each in turn. Common possibilities include:

- Changing washing powders etc. (particularly common with skin problems).
- Starting or stopping supplements, herbs and drugs, etc.
- Experiencing something psychologically stressful, etc.

For example, a client came back because her psoriasis had become worse. Muscle testing made it clear that she had started to do something new and that had caused the problem. She volunteered that she had started to take cod liver oil for her arthritis. Testing showed that this had caused her psoriasis to flare up again.

FINAL THOUGHTS

I practised kinesiology from 1982 to 2005. As well as allowing me to earn a living in such a satisfying way, it allowed me dramatically to improve the health of my two sons. My own health has responded too. Before I became a kinesiologist many people thought I was a hypochondriac because I was always complaining about one ailment or another. It brought my partner, John Payne, to me: first as a client, then as a student, then as someone to spend my life with.

I have seen many changes in the last twenty plus years, with kinesiology becoming more and more accepted. I have also seen many changes within kinesiologies, as practitioners, teachers and students begin to recognise the commonality that we share through these remarkable tools.

I hope this book will contribute to your professional growth, and that it will inspire you respectfully, but eagerly, to use the verbal questioning skills taught in this book to help yourself, your loved ones and your clients to better health, greater happiness and a more comprehensive expression of potential.

APPENDIX 1: PHYSICAL BODY SYSTEMS

- Cardiovascular (circulation + heart)
- Digestive
- Endocrine
- Integumentary (skin)
- Lymphatic
- Muscular & Connective Tissue
- Nervous
- Reproductive
- Respiratory
- Sensory (touch, pain, taste, sight, smell, hearing, equilibrium)
- Skeletal
- Urinary

APPENDIX 2: GRAMMAR

For our purposes word types can be usefully divided into:

- Nouns
- Pronouns
- Verbs
- Adjectives
- Adverbs
- Prepositions
- Determiners
- Conjunctions
- Interjections

Nouns

Words that are the names of things (concrete or abstract)
e.g. being a perfect *person*; accepting *success;* I like *chocolate*.

Two important sub-categories:

- **Proper nouns**: these are words that are the names of specific people, places, times, etc. and are written starting with a capital letter, e.g. loving *Peter*; waiting until *February* to see *Mary* in *London*.
- **Gerunds**: these are based on verbs, always end in –ing, and act like nouns, e.g. *feeling* happy (this looks like a verb, but, it is a truncated sentence).

Pronouns

Words that stand for a noun or a whole noun phrase, e.g. giving *him* the love *he* needs; knowing that *it*'s O.K. ; giving *myself* love; knowing the future is *mine*, etc.

Useful sub-categories are:

- **Personal pronouns**: e.g. I, me, myself, we, him, etc.
- **Possessive Pronouns**: e.g. mine, theirs, his, etc. (without a noun afterwards), e.g. this is *mine*.
- **Relative pronouns**: e.g. who, whom, whose, which, etc. e.g. being the person *who* others respect.
- **Indefinite pronouns**: e.g. someone, anyone, no one, somebody, all, each, none, few, etc.
- **Interrogative pronouns**: e.g. why, when, who, etc used in questions.
- e.g. *who* is that?

Verbs

Words which express a wide range of meanings, such as actions, sensations or states of being.
e.g. *to be* happy; I *can live* on my own.

There are several sub-categories:

- **Primary verbs**: be, have and do, e.g. accepting what I *have* to accept.
- **Modal verbs:** verbs such as will, can, could, shall, may, might, would, should, ought to, need to, have to, must, e.g. I *should* be happy.
- **Action verbs:** to run, to go, to stay
- **State verbs:** to appear, to seem, to see

For **gerunds** see the section on nouns.

Adjectives

Words which express some feature or quality of a noun or pronoun; they describe the noun, e.g. feeling *clever*; being the *best* student; accepting *critical* remarks, *imagined* worries.
Verbs can be used as adjectives e.g. a *frightened* woman, this film is *frightening*.

Adverbs

Words that often (but not always) end in -ly. They modify a word or phrase, most often an adjective, a verb or another adverb, e.g. being *totally* exhausted; working *hard* (hard can also be an adjective as in "a hard bed"); knowing *nearly* everything; wanting to give myself *totally* to God; accepting I can *always* change.

There are two main sub-categories:
- **Adverbs of frequency**: always, never, sometimes, now, occasionally, frequently, etc.
- **Adverbs of manner**: describe how something is done e.g. carelessly, beautifully, slowly, etc.

Prepositions

Words that express a relationship of meaning between two parts of a sentence. They most often show how the two parts are related in space or time, e.g. being *at* home; living *with* Tina.

Useful sub-categories are:

- **Prepositions of space**: e.g. between, above, on, into, near, beside, along, below, etc.
- **Prepositions of time:** e.g. until, since, past, before, after, at, during, etc.
- **Prepositions of movement**: e.g. toward, towards, to.
- **Verb + preposition**: e.g. look up to, work for, etc.

- **Adjective + preposition**: e.g. fond of, similar to, etc.
- **Noun + preposition**: e.g. concern for, participation in, etc.

Here is a fairly comprehensive list of prepositions:

About
Above
According to
Across
Adjacent to
After
Against
Along
Among
Amongst
Around
At
Before
Behind
Below
Beneath
Beside
Besides
Between
Betwixt
Beyond
By
By way of
Down
During
Except
For
From
In
In addition to
In front of
In place of

In regard to
In spite of
In the midst of
Inside
Instead of
Into
Like
More than
Near
Next to
Of
Off
On
On account of
Opposite to
Other than
Out of
Outside
Over
Past
Since
Through
Throughout
Till
To
Toward
Towards
Under
Underneath
Until
Up
Up to
Upon
Via
With
Within
Without

Determiners

Words such as a, the, some, each, few and those, which precede nouns, e.g. being *the* best student; giving myself *some* time; accepting *this* life (in the phrase "accepting *this*" the word this is a pronoun because it is not followed by a noun).

A fairly comprehensive list of determiners:

all
an
any
both
each
enough
every
few
latter
last
many
next
no
previous
several
some
subsequent
that
the
this
those
whatever
whichever

also numbers (one, two, one hundred etc.)
also ordinal numerals (first, second, hundredth)

Conjunctions

Words that join parts of a sentence together e.g. but, and, if, or, as, when, etc., e.g. I like to be on my own, *when* I want to read a book.

Interjections

Words used to exclaim, protest or command, e.g. wow, oh, no, yes, etc. e.g. *No*, don't do that! *Oh*, I forgot to tell you.

References For The Grammar Section:

Rediscover Grammar by David Crystal ISBN 0 582 00258 3
http://ccc.commnet.edu/grammar/
http://www.thebeehive.org/external_link.asp?r=/school/middle/subj
ects.asp?subject=12&e=http://www.dailygrammar.com/archive.sht
ml
Additional help from Giulia Boden and Stephanie Robertson

APPENDIX 3: FOOD CATEGORISATION

I usually use culinary categories and food families when testing for allergies and intolerances, and all three categories when testing for beneficial foods.

Culinary Categories

- Meat
- Fish
- Dairy
- Chicken and eggs
- Vegetables
- Herbs
- Pulses
- Pasta and rice
- Fruit
- Seeds and nuts
- Oils and fats
- Spices
- Bread, cakes
- Processed food

Nutritional Categories

- Proteins / amino acids
- Fats
- Carbohydrate
- Vitamins
- Minerals

Food Families

This is not a totally comprehensive list but covers most of the commonly eaten foods:

Banana
Banana, plantain

Birch
Filbert, hazelnut

Buckwheat
Buckwheat, garden sorrel, rhubarb

Cashew
Cashew nut, mango, pistachio (also poison ivy)

Citrus
Orange, lemon, grapefruit, tangerine, clementine, ugly fruit, satsuma, lime, angostura, kumquat, mandarin

Composite
Lettuce, chicory, sesame, sunflower, safflower, burdock, dandelion, camomile, artichoke (globe and Jerusalem), pyrethrum, absinthe, salsify, vermouth, ragweed, yarrow, endive

Euphorbia
Cassava, tapioca

Fungi Or Moulds
Baker's yeast, brewer's yeast, mushroom, truffle, chanterelle, blue cheese, vinegar, antibiotics

Gooseberry
Red currant, black currant, gooseberry

Goosefoot
Spinach, chard, sugar beet, lamb's lettuce / quarters, thistle, beetroot

Gourd
Melon, cucumber, squash, gherkin, courgette, marrow, pumpkin

Grape
Wine, champagne, brandy, sherry, raisin, currant (dried), sultana, cream of tartar, wine vinegar

Grasses
Wheat, corn, barley, oats, millet, cane sugar, bamboo shoots, rice, rye (note that buckwheat is *not* a member of the grass family)

Heath
Cranberry, blueberry, huckleberry, wintergreen

Laurel
Avocado, bay, camphor, cinnamon, laurel, sassafras

Legume / Pulses
Acacia, alfalfa, gum Arabic, pea, carob, cassia, chick pea, green bean, guar gum, haricot bean, kidney bean, lentil, liquorice, lima bean, locust bean gum, mung bean, navy bean, peanut, pinto bean, soya bean, textured vegetable protein (TVP), string bean, tamarind, tragacanth gum, urd flour (used in Indian cookery)

Lily
Onion, asparagus, chives, leek, garlic, sarsaparilla, shallot

Mallow
Cottonseed, okra

Mint
Mint, peppermint, basil, marjoram, oregano, sage, rosemary, savoury, thyme, balm

Morning Glory
Sweet potato, yam

Mulberry
Breadfruit, fig, hops, mulberry

Mustard
Broccoli, cabbage, cauliflower, Brussels sprouts, collard, horse-radish, kohlrabi, radish, swede, turnip, watercress, mustard, cress, watercress, rutabaga, kale

Myrtle
Allspice, cloves, eucalyptus, guava

Nightshade
Potato, tomato, tobacco, aubergine/eggplant, cayenne, bell pepper, chilli, sweet pepper, paprika, pimento

Nutmeg
Mace, nutmeg, brazil nut

Palm
Coconut, date, sago
Parsley
Carrot, parsley, dill, celery, fennel, parsnip, aniseed, angelica, celeriac, caraway, coriander, cumin, sweet cicely

Pulses Or Legumes
Pea, chick pea, soy bean (hence TVP), lentils, liquorice, peanut, kidney bean, string bean, haricot bean, mung bean, alfalfa

Rose
Apple, pear, quince, almond, apricot, cherry, peach, plum, sloe, blackberry, loganberry, raspberry, strawberry, boysenberry, dewberry, nectarine, prune, bilberry, blueberry, huckleberry, cranberry (this family is sometimes sub-divided further)

Sterculia
Chocolate, cocoa, cola nut

Walnut
Walnut, pecan, butternut, hickory

There appear to be several different ways of classifying animals. Here is one possibility.

Ruminants
Cattle (beef), milk and dairy products, mutton, lamb, goat, deer (venison)

Duck
Duck, goose

Game Birds
Pheasant, quail, turkey (turkey also gets listed under poultry)

Poultry
Chicken, eggs, turkey (turkey also gets listed under game birds)

Swine
Pork, bacon, lard (dripping), ham, sausage

Codfish
Haddock, cod, ling (saith), coley, hake

Crustaceans
Lobster, prawn, shrimp, crab, crayfish

Flatfish
Dab, flounder, halibut, turbot, sole, plaice

Herring
Pilchard, sardine, herring, rollmop

Mackerel
Tuna, bonito, tuny, mackerel, skipjack

Molluscs
Snail, abalone, squid, clam, mussel, oyster, scallop

Salmon
Salmon, trout, bass, catfish, perch, pike

The following foods have no *commonly* eaten relatives:

> juniper, pineapple, vanilla, black pepper, chestnut, maple, lychee, kiwi fruit, tea, coffee, papaya, ginseng, olive anchovy, sturgeon (caviar), rabbit

APPENDIX 4: EMOTIONS

This is a list of ten different basic emotions with words that I categorise under them. It is not meant to be totally comprehensive, nor is it the only way you can classify emotions.

The words have been expressed here as adjectives, but could equally well be used as nouns or adverbs.

The basic emotions are:

Anger
Fear
Sadness
Apathy
Lust
Pride
Bravery
Love
Happiness
Peace

ANGER

Abrasive
Abhorrent
Abusive
Acrimonious
Aggressive
Aggrieved
Angry
Annoyed
Antagonistic
Antagonized
Argumentative
Belligerent
Bitchy
Bitter
Boisterous
Brutal
Bugged
Bullying
Burning
Caustic
Chaotic
Choleric
Cranky
Cross
Cruel
Cynical
Destructive
Defensive
Defiant
Demanding
Destructive
Disgusted Displeased
Enraged
Exasperated

Explosive
Fed-up
Ferocious
Fierce
Fiery
Forceful
Frustrated
Fuming
Furious
Gruff
Grumpy
Hard
Harsh
Hated
Heartless
Hostile
Hot-headed
Hot-tempered
Impatient
Ill humoured
Ill tempered
Incandescent
Incensed
Indignant
Inflamed
Infuriated
Inhuman
Insensitive
Insulted
Irascible
Irate
Irritable
Irritated
Jealous

Livid
Mad
Malevolent
Mean
Merciless
Murderous
Offended
On fire
Out of sorts
Outraged
Peevish
Petulant
Piqued
Pissed off
Pissed (American usage)
Pushy
Upset
Pitiless
Provoked
Quarrelsome
Raging
Raving
Rebellious
Resentful
Resistant
Revolted
Riled
Rough
Rude
Ruthless
Sabotaging
Sadistic
Sarcastic
Savage
Seething
Severe
Sharp
Simmering
Smouldering

Spiteful
Steely
Stern
Stubborn
Sulky
Sullen
Unkind
Unrelenting
Up in arms
Resentful
Vehement
Vengeful
Vicious
Violent
Wicked
Wild
Wilful
Wrathful

Fear

Afraid
Alarmed
Anxious
Apprehensive
Ashamed
Awed
Baffled
Bashful
Bewildered
Bothered
Careful
Cautious
Clammy
Concerned
Conflicted
Confused
Cowardly
Cowed
Cowering
Cringing
Daunted
Defensive
Degraded
Dismayed
Dissatisfied
Distraught
Distressed
Distrustful
Disturbed
Doubtful
Dread
Edgy
Embarrassed
Evasive
Faint-hearted

Fearful
Foreboding
Frantic
Frightened
Guilty
Hesitant
Horrified
Hot and bothered
Humiliated
Hysterical
Ill at ease
In suspense
In turmoil
Inhibited
Insecure
Intimidated
Irrational
Miserable
Mixed-up
Nervous
Neurotic
On edge
On tenterhooks
Overwrought
Panicky
Panic-stricken
Paralysed
Paranoid
Perplexed
Perturbed
Petrified
Phobic
Puzzled
Reluctant
Restless

Scared
Shaky
Shocked
Shy
Skulking
Stressed
Tormented
Torn
Trapped
Trembling
Troubled
Uncertain
Uncomfortable
Uneasy
Upset
Vulnerable
Wary
Weak
Worried
Yellow

Superstitious
Suspicious
Tense
Terrified
Threatened
Timid

Sadness

Abandoned
Abject
Abused
Anguished
Upset
Apologetic
Bad
Bereaved
Betrayed
Bleak
Blue
Broken hearted
Burdened
Cheated
Dark
Dejected
Desolate
Despairing
Desperate
Despondent
Disappointed
Disconsolate
Discontented
Discounted
Disgruntled
Disheartened
Distraught
Dismal
Dispirited
Displeased
Dissatisfied
Doleful
Down
Downcast
Downhearted

Forlorn
Gloomy
Glum
Grey
Grief-stricken
Grieving
Grim
Guilty
Heart broken
Heavy
Heavy-hearted
Hurt
In despair
In the dumps
Inadequate
Inconsolable
Inept
Insignificant
Joyless
Left out
Lonely
Longing
Martyred
Regretful
Melancholic
Miserable
Morose
Mournful
Needy
Oppressed
Pathetic
Pensive
Pitiable
Pitiful
Regretful

Rejected
Remorseful
Sad
Sombre
Sorrowful
Undeserving
Unfortunate
Unhappy
Unloved
Unpleasant
Unsmiling
Unwanted
Upset
Vulnerable
Wistful
Woebegone
Wounded
Wretched

Sorry
Suicidal
Tearful
Tormented
Tortured

Apathy

Alienated
Alone
Bored
Cold
Cool
Cut off
Dead
Defeated
Depressed
Demoralised
Discouraged
Disillusioned
Doomed
Drained
Emotionless
Empty
Helpless
Hopeless
Impassive
Inattentive
Indifferent
Unemotional
Unfeeling
Unfocussed
Uninterested
Unmoved
Unresponsive
Useless
Vague
Worthless

Introverted
Lazy
Listless
Lost
Low
Negative
Numb
Overwhelmed
Passive
Pessimistic
Phlegmatic
Pointless
Powerless
Resigned
Self-defeating
Spaced out
Spacey
Stoned
Stuck
Sullen
Tired

Lust

Ardent
Carnal
Compulsive
Craving
Demanding
Driven
Envious
Fixated
Frustrated
Gluttonous
Greedy
Hungry
Impatient
Lascivious
Lecherous
Libidinous
Licentious
Lustful
Manipulative
Miserly
Obsessed
Over indulgent
Passionate
Possessive
Predatory
Pushy
Randy
Raunchy
Reckless
Scheming
Selfish
Sensual
Sexy
Voracious

Wanton
Wicked

Pride

Aloof
Arrogant
Bigoted
Boastful
Clever
Closed
Complacent
Conceited
Contemptuous
Critical
Disdainful
Dogmatic
Egotistical
Gloating
Haughty
Hypocritical
Icy
Imperious
Inflexible
Isolated
Judgemental
Narrow-minded
Opinionated
Overbearing
Patronising
Pious
Prejudiced
Proud
Righteous
Rigid
Self important
Self satisfied
Selfish
Smug
Snobbish
Snooty

Special
Stoical
Stubborn
Stuck up
Supercilious
Superior
Uncompromising
Unforgiving
Unyielding
Vain

Bravery

Adventurous
Alert
Alive
Anticipating
Assured
Aware
Bold
Brave
Capable
Centred
Certain
Competent
Confident
Creative
Courageous
Daring
Decisive
Determined
Dynamic
Eager
Enthusiastic
Excited
Exhilarated
Exuberant
Fearless
Flexible
Focussed
Gallant
Heroic
Honourable
Independent
Inspired
Intrepid
Invincible

Motivated
Optimistic
Plucky
Positive
Purposeful
Resilient
Resolute
Secure
Self-sufficient
Strong
Sure
Tireless
Undaunted
Valiant
Vigorous
Visionary
Willing
Zealous

Love

Accepted
Accepting
Adored
Adoring
Affectionate
Amiable
Appreciated
Appreciative
Aroused
Cared for
Caressed
Caring
Cherished
Cherishing
Comforted
Compassionate
Connected
Consoled
Consoling
Doting
Embraced
Enchanted
Esteemed
Friendly
Gentle
Helpful
Included
Including
Intimate
Liked
Lovable
Loved
Lovely
Loving
Needed

Nurtured
Nurturing
Obsessed
Respected
Savoured
Smitten
Sociable
Tender
Warm
Welcoming

Happiness

Affable
Agreeable
Alert
Alive
Amiable
Amused
Animated
Anticipating
Appreciated
Blessed
Blissful
Blithe
Carefree
Charming
Cheerful
Comfortable
Congenial
Content
Contented
Delighted
Eager
Ecstatic
Elated
Encouraged
Enthusiastic
Excited
Exhilarated
Exuberant
Floating on air
Full of life
Gay
Glad
Glowing
Good-humoured
Good-natured

Gratified
Happy
Happy-go-lucky
Hopeful
Jolly
Joyful
Joyous
Jubilant
Kind
Kindly
Laughing
Light-hearted
Lively
Merry
Nonchalant
On cloud nine
Optimistic
Overjoyed
Over the moon
Patient
Playful
Pleasant
Pleased
Radiant
Rapt
Relieved
Satisfied
Sparkling
Sunny
Sure
Sweet
Sweet-tempered
Thrilled
Vibrant
Vital

Vivacious
Worthy

Peace

Abundant
Amicable
At ease
At peace
Balanced
Beautiful
Benevolent
Benign
Calm
Easy
Easy-going
Harmonious
Intuitive
Light
Mellow
Peaceful
Placid
Quiet
Relaxed
Restful
Serene
Still
Tranquil
Unconcerned
Undisturbed
Unruffled
Untroubled

LaVergne, TN USA
06 May 2010
181812LV00001B/6/P